# Living with Illness

## Psychosocial Challenges for Nursing

# Living with Illness

## Psychosocial Challenges for Nursing

**Edited by**

Cath **Rogers-Clark**
Alexandra **McCarthy**
Kristine **Martin-McDonald**

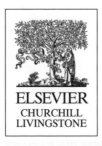

**ELSEVIER**
CHURCHILL
LIVINGSTONE

Sydney  Edinburgh  London  New York  Philadelphia  St Louis  Toronto

## ELSEVIER

Churchill Livingstone
is an imprint of Elsevier

Elsevier Australia
30-52 Smidmore Street, Marrickville, NSW 2204

*National Library of Australia Cataloguing-in-Publication Data*

---

Rogers-Clark, Cath.
 Living with illness : psychosocial challenges for nursing.

 Includes index.
 ISBN 0 7295 3750 1.

 1. Nursing.  2. Nursing - Social aspects.  3. Nursing -
 Psychological aspects.  I. Title.

610.73

---

Publisher: Vaughn Curtis
Publishing services manager: Helena Klijn
Project coordinator: Emma Hutchinson
Editor, project manager and proofreader: Persimmon Press
Cover and internal designer: Design Animals
Typesetter: Midland Typesetters Pty Ltd
Indexer: Max McMaster
Printed and bound in Australia by Ligare

# Foreword

People generally become nurses because they like people and want to help them. The profession of nursing allows this altruistic impulse to be harnessed into holistic care. The ability to provide holistic care is dependent upon knowing how to provide physical and psychosocial care, frequently simultaneously. It is the psychosocial aspects of nursing that nurses generally find to be the most challenging and rewarding parts of their work. Every day, at all hours of the day, nurses face complex psychosocial situations that require knowledge, skill and sensitivity to manage effectively. Most of these situations need to be responded to as they are unfolding; only rarely will the situation wait for a social worker or psychologist appointment during standard business hours. The task for nursing educators has been to try to ensure that students have a useable theoretical foundation in psychosocial aspects of care so that they have the essential knowledge needed to respond appropriately to people's complex and often painful psychosocial challenges.

This book marks a milestone in nursing's theoretical 'coming of age' in that the authors have creatively re-conceptualised knowledge from other disciplines including psychology, sociology and epidemiology. Previous works have exclusively used psychological concepts such as 'depression' and 'anxiety' or sociological concepts such as 'sick role' and 'capitalism' and student nurses, with little or no knowledge of nursing practice, have been expected to somehow integrate what they were being presented into their developing nursing knowledge base. Not surprisingly, many students found that difficult and questioned the relevance of being taught these subjects. Now the work of integration has been done for them making the whole subject much more relevant to practice and therefore easier to learn. Along with using some standard concepts such as 'class' and 'gender', the authors have extensively used nursing concepts which integrate the essential ideas from related disciplines into nursing in such a way that a new synthesis has been created. This has happened through the authors' use of nursing concepts such as health, illness, wellness, grieving, suffering, resilience, healing, cultural safety, spiritual wellbeing and holism.

This is a contemporary publication that canvasses the traditional areas of psychosocial knowledge and explores new areas of growing importance within the health care industry. New areas include men's health considered within gender and health, constructions of chronic illness, ageing, rural and remote peoples, illness and recovery as a journey. The final chapter, on empowering partnerships, provides a clear theoretical framework for nurses to use when they intervene to strengthen the social support networks of people living with illness. Readers will be delighted with the real life stories that are used to situate the ideas of psychosocial nursing within nursing practice.

*Professor Kathleen Fahy*
*Dean, School of Nursing & Midwifery*
*The University of Newcastle*

# Contents

# Contributors

**Lenore Beddoes**, MA Ed, BN (Hons), BsocSc, ITU Cert., DipCompN, RN, is currently a Lecturer in the School of Nursing, Deakin University, Victoria. She has a diverse clinical nursing background that includes medical, haematology, and surgical nursing with specialist experience in neurology and general intensive care. Lenore enjoys teaching, researching and writing about her special interest area of nursing across the acute-chronic interface.

**Odette Best** is a Punthamurra Gorreng/Gorreng woman who was born and raised in Brisbane and is currently employed as a nurse academic in the Department of Nursing, University of Southern Queensland. Odette is a hospital trained Registered Nurse, holds a Bachelor of Health Science undergraduate degree and a Master of Philosophy and is currently enrolled in her PhD. Odette has worked in Indigenous health for over twelve years and her passion is to see the integration of Indigenous health as core curriculum across all health disciplines.

**Elizabeth Bruce**, PhD MAPS, completed her doctorate in psychology at LaTrobe University, Victoria. Research into the nature of grief for individuals with chronic conditions formed the focus of this doctoral research. Elizabeth continues to offer training, consulting, therapeutic groupwork and clinical practice in this field. She is published in international and national journals. With her co-author, Dr Cynthia Schultz, she has recently written two texts, *Nonfinite loss and grief: A psychoeducational approach* (Elsevier, Sydney) and *Through Loss* (ACER, Melbourne).

**Colleen Cartwright** is a Senior Research Fellow in the Academic Unit in Geriatric Medicine in the School of Medicine, University of Queensland. She has an Honours Degree in Social Work, a Master of Public Health, and a PhD. Colleen assisted with the development and implementation of the Queensland *Powers of Attorney Act*, including designing the Advance Health Directive and Enduring Power of Attorney documents. She is Chief Investigator on the Australian arm of a major international research project into Medical Decisions at the End-of-Life.

**Don Gorman**, RN(EndMH), DipNEd, BEd, MEd, EdD, FANZCMHN, FRACN, is currently Associate Professor of Mental Health Nursing at the University of Southern Queensland. His major area of interest is in cross-cultural health care and education as exemplified by culture related research including healthy sexuality in long-term aged care in Australia and Spain, a collaborative model to address NIDDM in Indigenous Australian communities, and young Non-English speaking background people and mental health in South Australia, Western Australia and Queensland.

**Jan Horsfall**, RN, BA(Hons) (UNSW), MA(Hons) (UNE), PhD (La Trobe), is a recently retired academic. She has taught mental health nursing, research, sociology, and cross-cultural aspects of nursing for eighteen years at Charles Sturt University, LaTrobe University Bendigo, The University of Sydney and

The University of Western Sydney. Recent collaborative research projects include mental health nursing students' clinical learning; consumer involvement in practice change in mental health settings; and social capital among younger women in a low socioeconomic status Sydney suburb.

**Wendy Lee Kyle**, RN, BN, Dip T Teach, MN, began work as a clinical nurse in 1966 and has worked as a nurse manager and educator in Australia and New Zealand. She has a wide range of nursing experiences in health care and taught in the area of health and wellness and the psychosocial aspects of nursing including men's health. She is currently a lecturer at the University of Southern Queensland.

**Alexandra McCarthy** has worked as a clinician, educator and researcher in nursing since 1995. She is currently a member of the research committee of the Cancer Nurses Society of Australia and editorial board member of the Australian Journal of Cancer Nursing. She has a particular interest in pain management, and the longer-term outcomes of surviving both cancer and renal failure. Her PhD explored the historical constructions of breast cancer.

**Kristine Martin-McDonald**, RN, BAppSc, MEd, PhD, is an Associate Professor in the Faculty of Nursing at the University of Alberta, Edmonton, Canada. She teaches research courses to both undergraduate and postgraduate students and psychosocial nursing to undergraduates. Kristine's research is focused on Renal Replacement Therapies and Narrative Methodology.

**Victoria Parker**, RN, BHSc, Grad Dip Critical Care, MN, MRCNA, currently teaches in the Department of Nursing, University of Southern Queensland. Victoria has a broad background in nursing but predominantly critical care environments where she has significant experience in the teaching and education of nurses. Her research interests include aspects of cardiac rehabilitation looking particularly at the benefits for the ageing population.

**Cath Rogers-Clark**, RN, BA (Behavioural Science, with distinction), MN, PhD, is a Senior Lecturer in the Department of Nursing at the University of Southern Queensland. She teaches psychosocial nursing to undergraduate nursing students, and is currently supervising a number of Masters and PhD students in the area of women's health. Her own research is focused on women's responses to living with adversity, such as the long-term sequelae of cancer and its treatment.

**Cynthia Schultz** earned her doctorate in psychology from the University of Queensland and, as Senior Lecturer in the Faculty of Health Sciences, La Trobe University, taught in the areas of interpersonal skills, family dynamics, group processes, and loss and grief. Her research, publications, and community involvements have focused on caregiving issues and loss and grief. She was foundation editor of the *Journal of Family Studies*. Now a freelance academic, enjoying creative retirement, she focuses on extending her earlier work, the most recent example of which is co-authorship with Dr Elizabeth Bruce of *Through Loss*, published in 2004 by ACER Press.

**Noel C Schultz**, BA, MA, DMin, is a minister of the Uniting Church now in active retirement. He has co-authored five books with Dr Cynthia Schultz and two national psychoeducational group programs of support for carers (*Caring for Family Caregivers* and *Care for Caring Parents*). In his appointment as Coordinator of Ministry with Older Adults in the Synod of Victoria and Tasmania, he emphasised the ongoing role of older people in the life of churches and communities, working to strengthen the spiritual care of persons with dementia and their carers. His most recent work is the 2004 book, *Forgetting but not forgotten: Understanding, support, and spiritual care of persons with dementia and their carers* (OpenBook, Adelaide).

**Bev Taylor**, RN, RM, MEd, PhD, is the Foundation Chair in Nursing in the School of Nursing and Health Care Practices, Southern Cross University, Lismore, New South Wales. Bev is the author of many books and journal articles relating to nursing and health. She is the Research Director of the School of Nursing and Health Care Practices and the Editor of the *Australian Journal of Holistic Nursing*.

**Sally J Wellard**, PhD, MN, BA(Soc Sc), Renal Cert, RN, is Foundation Professor, School of Nursing, University of Ballarat. Dr Wellard has enjoyed a varied clinical nursing career including in surgical, community and renal care nursing. She enjoys teaching, conducting research and writing about chronic illness management, consumer participation in care and clinical education for nurses.

**Geoff Wilson**, RN Cardiothoracic Certificate, DNE, GD Advanced Clin Nsg (Emergency), Dip NEd, B AppSc (Advanced Nsg), MN, MCNA, has been extensively involved in critical care and health promotion in Australia and overseas, and was the founding director of a Cardiac Rehabilitation and Lifestyle Education Centre in Toowoomba. He is currently senior lecturer and Director of Clinical Schools at the University of Southern Queensland, teaching medical-surgical and critical care nursing. He maintains a practice interest in emergency nursing and critical care, and research interests in men's health, men in nursing and cardiac rehabilitation.

# Preface

This book is for undergraduate nursing students studying psychosocial foundation units, and practising nurses who seek to understand more about the illness experience.

Traditionally, nurses have drawn on knowledge from sociology and psychology—two separate but related disciplines to nursing—leaving the beginning level nurse to relate, integrate, translate and transfer that knowledge into nursing practice. In this text we have tried to combine socio-logical and psychological insights with nursing knowledge to present a psychosocial perspective that is innovative and directly applicable to contem-porary nursing practice.

After fifteen years of teaching psychology and sociology to nursing students, we believe we are at a time when psychosocial nursing research has come of age. Qualitative nursing research, in particular, has revealed rich insights into peoples' experiences of illness. Our intention has been to ensure that at least some of this work is captured within an introductory text that nursing students will find accessible and, hopefully, interesting and relevant. We were motivated primarily by our own teaching experiences. We had struggled to find texts for students in the psychosocial arena, given our preference for Australian content that is nursing based rather than emanating from the disciplines of psychology and sociology. This text is our attempt to fill this gap.

It has, as always, been a challenge to create this book. Many people have helped us realise our goal and, in particular, we acknowledge the work of our chapter contributors, who willingly toiled to create their individual chapters. Each chapter then needed appropriate revisions to ensure we created a single, cohesive text, rather than a series of unrelated chapters.

We would also like to thank the staff of Elsevier for their support, namely Vaughn Curtis and Rhiain Hull for their ever-prompt and professional attention to us. We were also blessed with the support of three dedicated book reviewers who gave of their valuable time to carefully read the first draft of this book and provide excellent feedback that helped us complete our final edit of the text. We have also valued the support of our editor, Alison Moodie, whose standard of work is in our opinion quite exceptional.

We'd also like to acknowledge the many hundreds of students we have taught and who have taught us more than they could ever realise. Indeed, it was our experiences with students that formed the genesis of this text, and their contribution to our knowledge and understanding of what students need in a psychosocial nursing course is in no small way reflected in the approach, content and structure of this book.

Finally, we thank our long-suffering families for their patience and forbearance during the creation of this book. There have been stressful times, but we think the book is worth the effort.

We do hope that you enjoy the book and find it relevant to your practice. It's easy to forget the psychosocial needs of patients in the rush to become

## Preface

'technically competent', but psychosocial knowledge and skills are fundamental to nursing practice and, indeed, are recognised as core competencies of the beginning registered nurse by the Australian Nursing Council. We hope that this book is a valuable tool in helping you think more deeply about your patients' experiences, and hence provide nursing care that is sensitive to the holistic needs of all those you care for.

*Cath Rogers-Clark, Alexandra McCarthy and*
*Kristine Martin-McDonald, July 2004*

# Chapter 1

## Introduction to Psychosocial Nursing

*Cath Rogers-Clark*

**This chapter:**

- defines psychosocial nursing care;
- explores evidence supporting the value of high quality psychosocial care; and
- introduces the chapters in this text.

This textbook is for nurses interested in providing a high quality service for their clients who are challenged by illness. Responding to psychosocial needs is an essential aspect of health care and, together with good physical care, provides for the needs of individuals, families and groups accessing health care. The book is aimed at undergraduate students studying psychosocial foundation units, and practising nurses who seek to understand more about the illness experience. Its focus is on developing and strengthening the empathic insight of readers, critically appraising conventional approaches to understanding and caring for those who are ill, and empowering readers to offer true holistic care using, where possible, evidence-based practice.

As a student within a health-related discipline, one of the critical areas of study is the study of people—whether as individuals, or as members of families, groups and communities. A deeper and more educated understanding and appreciation for all people is a quality which nurses must continually strive to develop if they wish to be effective in their caring role. Knowledge and technical competence often do not compensate for a lack of empathy for people experiencing illness and/or crises.

What is psychosocial care? Psychosocial care is any response from a health professional that helps people to deal with the social, cultural and psychological dimensions of their illness. Psychosocial care may also be extended to those coping with a life transition or crisis which is affecting their health and wellbeing (Gorman, Raines & Sultan 2002). In order to help, it is first necessary to understand the life world of the other; a challenge for nurses who may ordinarily have little time to listen, reflect and empathise due to pressures such as workload, time and resource constraints.

# Case study

Jenny is 49. After a routine mammogram, she was diagnosed with an aggressive form of breast cancer. This came as a huge shock to her. Within a week, she had the cancerous part of her breast and surrounding tissue removed. Once she had recovered a little from the surgery, she commenced chemotherapy. After six months of chemotherapy, she began seven weeks of radiotherapy. It was during this treatment that she spent time talking to the specialist breast care nurse (Anne). The specialist breast care nurse position had just been created in Jenny's town, which is in a regional area two hours drive from a major city. Jenny said it was a relief to finally talk to somebody. Anne spent two hours with her, just listening.

'I feel like I'm numb. I just don't feel anything. I'm walking around in a fog. I guess it's better that way. I can't tell you how bad it's been. I can't really believe I'm still alive. I thought I'd go mad. The chemo . . . I just vomited all the time. I lost my hair. I can't talk to my husband. I guess he cares about me, but he just can't communicate very well. I could talk to my daughters, but I don't want to worry them. They've been through enough already, what with me being diagnosed and all. Now they have to live with the worry that they might get breast cancer too. That's a great gift I've given them isn't it!'

'Everyone's been great . . . the doctors, nurses, X-ray people . . . I haven't met a bad one. I haven't really been able to talk much to them though. They're all so busy.'

There is substantial evidence that good quality psychosocial care makes a difference. For example, thirty years of research has confirmed that the provision of information, counselling and supportive care improves health outcomes and wellbeing for women with breast cancer (Redman, Turner & Davis 2003). In other words, good psychosocial care doesn't just make patients feel better emotionally; it can also influence their physical health! Despite this evidence, Redman et al (2003) note that many psychosocial interventions proven to be of worth have not been routinely adopted into clinical practice. This was the case with Jenny. She acknowledges that her physical care has been excellent and notes the kindness of all those nurses caring for her. And yet, she hasn't had the opportunity with any of these professionals to really talk about how she is feeling.

In one Australian study (Irurita 1999), patients identified many factors which affected whether they felt well cared for or not. These factors included environmental issues, such as perceptions of ageism from some nurses, lack of funding and related staffing levels, and early discharge policies. Organisational factors included the quality of services offered by the health service, such as quality of food, communication and coordination between the different caregivers, information to patients, consistency in caregivers, and time available and how this influenced the nurse–patient relationship. Finally, the personal qualities of each health professional were seen to influence the quality of care patients received. As one participant in Irurita's study noted (p 93), 'I think all of the staff are trained to a very high level, but the level of compassion varies.' In our case study, when Jenny finally got the opportunity to talk with Anne, the breast care nurse, Jenny not only received compassion but by being attentive, open and non-judgmental, the nurse empowered Jenny to share her experience and story in a manner that met Jenny's need at that time. Jenny felt very relieved that she could finally talk about her feelings.

A qualitative research project investigating nurses' perceptions of quality care revealed that the registered nurse participants saw psychosocial nursing as 'being there' in a supportive role (Williams 1998). Core skills in psychosocial nursing were seen to be communicating effectively, giving information, caring and being an advocate for the patient and family. A high level of care, termed therapeutically effective care by Williams, occurred when 'therapeutically conducive relationships' were established between nurses and their patients (1998 p 810). Trust and rapport were essential aspects of these relationships and evident in the case study relationship between Jenny and the nurse. The registered nurses who participated in William's study argued that therapeutically conducive relationships underpinned the provision of effective nursing care. That is, patients' needs could only be properly assessed once these relationships were established. Jenny may have been experiencing a sense of guilt for the burden that her illness had brought to her family, but this could only be identified and addressed after the establishment of a therapeutic relationship between Jenny and her nurses.

This book attempts to reveal the complexities that chronic illness brings to the lives of patients and their families as a way of encouraging nurses to empathetically connect with that illness experience.

## This book

Using a situated learning approach, this text utilises nursing, sociological and psychological theories to explore the psychosocial, spiritual and cultural needs of people requiring health care. Theory based on research evidence is applied to develop a deeper understanding of, and appreciation for, the needs of people from a variety of backgrounds who need individualised, sensitive health care during an episode of vulnerability. To help 'make sense' of relevant theory, this text incorporates case studies, to share the voices of those living with illness.

This book is divided into four sections. In the first section, Chapter 1 provides an introduction to the content, psychosocial focus and use of case studies throughout the book and highlights the focus of each chapter. In Chapter 2, Health, Wellness, Illness, Healing and Holism, and Nursing, Beverly Taylor introduces the concepts of the chapter title. These concepts form the basis for this text, and will be described in some depth in this chapter. The concept of holistic nursing is explored, and the ways in which nurses can be healing in their partnerships with patients are discussed. This chapter also focuses on 'emotional labour'; that is, nurses' use of emotional expression in their therapeutic relationships, as a means of engaging with, and assisting the health of, their patients and families.

In the second section (Chapters 3 to 8), the social contexts of illness experiences are explored. This focus acknowledges that an illness experience is always embedded in the social life of an individual, and the position of that person within their community. The third section (Chapters 9 to 12) moves on to consider specific aspects of illness experiences—suffering and resilience, pain and fatigue and loss and grief. Finally, in the last section (Chapter 13), the text concludes with a focus on the partnership model as an effective basis for offering psychosocial care to those who are ill.

In Chapter 3, Class, Poverty and Chronic Illness—Intersecting Links, Jan Horsfall presents the irrefutable evidence that links social class, poverty and illness. The terms 'class' and 'poverty' are defined and explored, and the intersection between socioeconomic status and health status explained. A social model of health, incorporating primary health principles, is presented as a framework for nurses and other health care professionals to most usefully address the social causes of ill health. A case study of a person living with cardiovascular disease is used to demonstrate how class is strongly associated with a higher risk of illness, and how class and poverty can strongly affect the illness experiences of a person with cardiovascular disease.

As a major source of division and inequality within society, gender has a powerful influence on health and illness experiences. In Chapter 4, Gender and Health, Cath Rogers-Clark, Wendy Lee Kyle and Geoff Wilson have written about the ways in which gender influences the patterns of health and illness which people experience, as well as their illness journeys and the responses they receive from nurses. A variety of perspectives on the health of women are explored, as well as the growing body of research examining men's health issues. Two case studies are used to explore the ways in which gender constructions influence both health and illness experiences, and the quality of health care provided.

As the populations of affluent nations age, the work of nurses is increasingly focused on caring for older persons. Colleen Cartwright and Victoria Parker note, in Chapter 5, Ageing in Health and Illness, that many older people accessing health care experience a range of chronic illnesses, which challenge their quality of life and require supportive and coordinated care from nurses and other health care providers. Regrettably, ageist beliefs can lead to health care provision marred by paternalistic practices. Whatever their health status, older people seek health care which begins with the premise that older people have the same needs for autonomy, respect and compassion as any other adult patient. This chapter alerts readers to the mythology surrounding older people, and encourages them to develop accurate perceptions of the experience of ageing, which encompasses positive as well as negative life changes. A case study of an older person living with arthritis is used to explore the vulnerabilities and resilience of older peoples in relation to their health and wellbeing.

In Chapter 6, Multicultural Issues in Health, written by Don Gorman and Odette Best, the cultural contexts of illness experiences are discussed. Health beliefs and practices vary from culture to culture, making cultural sensitivity essential to the delivery of effective health care. The chapter looks at the issues related to health care in a multicultural environment and the knowledge, attitudes and skills necessary to care for people from different cultures. It is particularly focused on the needs of nurses working with Australia's Indigenous peoples, as well as people who have migrated to Australia. A case study documenting the experiences of an Indigenous person confronting health difficulties is provided.

Around 30% of Australians live outside a major city. In Chapter 7, Health Issues for People in Rural and Remote Areas, Cath Rogers-Clark and Alexandra McCarthy explore the illness experiences of people living in rural and remote parts of Australia. In describing client-related psychosocial issues, the chapter explores the demographic challenges, the impact of the environment and cultural issues that influence clients' perceptions of illness and wellbeing. The chapter also explores the challenges that rural and remote nurses must meet to deliver quality psychosocial care in these areas. A case study examining a rural family's experiences of living through illness illustrates how a rural context can influence the health and wellbeing of rural residents.

The social meanings of chronic illness are explored in Chapter 8, Constructions of Chronic Illness, by Sally Wellard and Lenore Beddoes. This chapter describes major influences on biomedical and psychosocial approaches to understanding experiences of chronic illness, and critically reviews the effects of individualistic, scientific approaches to delivering health care to those with chronic illness. The concept of 'normalisation' is explored, and linked to the development of stigma in chronic illness. A case study of a young woman living with diabetes is used to illustrate how chronic illness is experienced.

Pain and fatigue can be the most overwhelming symptoms impairing quality of life for those living with an acute and chronic illness, but they are not easily amenable to medication-led approaches to illness management. Chapter 9 Living with Illness: Pain and Fatigue, written by Alexandra McCarthy, explores the psychosocial aspects of pain and fatigue. The characteristics of pain and fatigue are described, as well as a range of issues vital to accurately assessing pain and fatigue. This chapter moves on to consider how pain, fatigue, anxiety, depression and sleep dysfunction can become inter-related in those with chronic illness, and finally outlines interventions to assist those who experience pain and fatigue associated with chronic illness.

Loss is an integral part of life, and those who are unwell may confront a range of losses associated with their illness. Chapter 10, Living with Loss and Grief, is written by Cynthia Schultz and Elizabeth Bruce. They note that grieving is a traumatic but normal response to loss. It is a personal journey, and it is the role of the nurse to support each person as they travel through grief. A key aspect of this chapter will be an emphasis on debunking myths about grieving; for example that grieving proceeds in stages and that grieving should be completed within a given timeframe. Instead, readers are offered guidelines for supporting those who are living with loss, including anticipating and preparing for death and dying.

Illness has been likened to a journey by many authors as a way of reflecting the reality that there may be several pathways that are selected and traversed, with detours, delays, and obstacles overcome to reach a point where acceptance of a changed self and social world is established. Suffering is a profound and disturbing experience that is an actual or perceived threat to the integrity and social world of an individual. It is not restricted to physical assault, but incorporates cultural, spiritual, psychological and social ones as well. Chapter 11, Journeys Through Illness: Suffering and Resilience, written by Kristine Martin-McDonald and Cath Rogers-Clark, introduces the concepts of uncertainty, enduring, hope, resilience and survivorship as ways of understanding the capacity of people to move through the suffering associated with health-related adversity. This chapter moves on to discuss strategies that nurses will find helpful in assisting people to strengthen their resilient capacities as they journey through illness. A case study is used throughout to illustrate one person's experience of journeying through illness.

In Chapter 12, The Spiritual Dimension in Health Care, Reverend Noel Schultz considers the centrality of the spirit in the experience of being human. The concept of spirituality is defined, and the differences between religiosity and spirituality explored. The importance of spiritual wellbeing to those who confront health-related difficulties is discussed through a consideration of the spiritual needs of Mary, a woman with dementia. Key aspects of spiritual nursing care are highlighted and exemplified by the caring actions of Mary's nurses. This chapter acknowledges the challenges in providing spiritual nursing care, but notes that responding to a patient's spiritual needs involves a broad range of responses which may be no more burdensome than more traditional modes of providing nursing care.

The final chapter in this text, Chapter 13, Empowering Partnerships: Nurses and Those They Care For, written by Kristine Martin-McDonald, concludes that living with illness is a personal challenge for individuals and those who love them. There is clear evidence that positive social support is instrumental in maintaining and enhancing health and wellbeing. The capacity to respond well to the challenge of illness is likely to be enhanced by supportive care from nurses and other health workers. This chapter focuses on tangible, practical guidelines for nurses providing support to those living with acute and chronic illness. It emphasises the importance of 'being with' those who are suffering, and outlines the features of a partnership approach between nurses, patients and their families.

## Tutorial questions

1. What knowledge, skills and attributes do nurses need to be able to provide compassionate, holistic care?
2. What knowledge, skills and attributes do *you* need to develop before you feel competent to provide good psychosocial care?

## References

Gorman L, Raines M, Sultan D 2002 *Psychosocial nursing for general patient care*, 2nd edn. Davis, Philadelphia
Irurita V 1999 Factors affecting the quality of nursing care: The patient's perspective. *International Journal of Nursing Practice* 5:86–94

Redman S, Turner J, Davis C 2003 Improving supportive care for women with breast cancer in Australia: the challenge of modifying health systems. *Psycho-Oncology* 12:521–531

Williams A 1998 The delivery of quality nursing care: a grounded theory study of the nurse's perspective. *Journal of Advanced Nursing* 27:808–816

# Chapter 2

## Health, Wellness, Illness, Healing and Holism, and Nursing

*Beverley Taylor*

**This chapter:**

- explores the concepts of health, wellness, illness, healing, holism and holistic nursing;
- discusses ways in which nurses can develop healing partnerships with those they care for; and
- identifies how nurses' use of emotional expression can facilitate their healing work.

This chapter introduces the concepts of health, wellness, illness, healing and holism. These concepts form the basis for this text, and hence are described in some depth. The concept of holistic nursing is explored, and the ways in which nurses can be healing in their partnerships with patients are discussed. This chapter also focuses on 'emotional labour' in nursing; that is, nurses' use of emotional expression in their therapeutic relationships as a means of engaging with, and assisting the health of, their patients and families. The ideas inherent within the concept of health, wellness, illness, healing and holism, 'emotional labour' and therapeutic relationships apply to nurses whose work centres on human interactions.

## Health

This section deals with definitions of health from the accepted World Health Organization (WHO) definition and critiques of its shortcomings from an Indigenous Australian perspective. Also considered is the nature of a 'health promoting hospital'. Many attempts have been made to define human health (for example, Bright 2002, Smith 2002, Thompson 2002), and it may seem strange that such a simple word could cause so much debate. In the light of differing opinions, nurses and caring professionals may resort to the World Health Organization definition that has gained increasing acceptance, that 'health is a state of complete physical, mental and social wellbeing and not merely the absence of disease or infirmity' (WHO 1974, p 1). While this definition of health seems reasonable, because it is from a reputable source and it encompasses a holistic view, it has been criticised for being more closely applied to happiness than to health, thus having no practical use (Saracci 1997) and for failing 'to capture the dynamic or *action-oriented* nature of being healthy and well' (McMurray 2003, p 9).

Saracci's argument is that the WHO definition of health of inherent completeness corresponds most closely with the notion of happiness when individuals are seen to be healthier and happier (1997, p 1409). His contention is that health and happiness do not necessarily increase in the same direction and that it is possible to be healthier, say from stopping smoking, but to be a lot less happy as a result. He goes on to argue that happiness is subjective and elusive, particular only to how it is felt and interpreted subjectively by an individual, whereas health is a 'positive and universal human right'. He suggests a better descriptor would be that 'health is a condition of well being free of disease or infirmity and a basic human right' (1997, p 1410).

McMurray (2003, p 9) applauds the WHO's attempt to incorporate 'physical, psychological, cultural and social factors' in their definition of health, but she claims that it does not represent health as a dynamic phenomenon. Her contention is that 'health is not always experienced as the ideal described above'; rather, it is relative to the person, changing with individual 'circumstances, context and perceptions'. She suggests that we consider 'individual perspectives on health, or the extent to which people define themselves as healthy' and offers examples of people who consider themselves healthy, even though they may have a disability, or be recovering from surgery, illness or injury. She makes the point that people interpret adversity and limitations differently and, while some people may see themselves in terms of their disability others may use their disability as a challenge to excel in their lives and to 'achieve higher levels of health than they had previously experienced' (McMurray 2003, p 10).

However, other definitions of health far extend the WHO's parameters. For example, consider an Australian Aboriginal perspective on holistic health (Warrawee'a 2000, p 6), that:

> . . . your health is utterly dependent on the health of *all* things—tangible and intangible, ponderable and imponderable. All life, matter, and energy is one united entity of which we are an inseparable part; and that to treat any *single* part is insufficient to bring about the totality of health.

The nature of holism in this definition considers all life, matter and energy, including humans as one, thus rejecting separateness and singularity. Therefore, it is possible to not only to consider differing perspectives of health, but to also to contemplate different degrees of holism, ranging from a combination of parts to an inseparable mass of oneness, depending on the perspective with which you resonate. There will be further discussion on holism later in this chapter.

## Case study

As a young child, Andrew was diagnosed with asthma and often missed out on sports events because he was ill. After an acute admission to hospital, when Andrew was 13 years old, an asthma nurse educator discussed different management options with Andrew and his parents. Andrew was keen to begin self-management and really got interested in learning as much as he could about his disease and strategies for managing it. Whilst the parents were initially reluctant, they were encouraged by the nurse indicating that a health promotion focus, with Andrew self-managing, could lead to a better quality of life.

Given that health is a right for all people, it is promoted actively at individual, community, global and universal levels. Andrew's ability to manage his asthma created a sense of wellness and confidence in him as he was setting and achieving goals that were important to him. As health increases feelings of wellness and predictions of life expectancy, it gives quality to those years. A change in the focus of hospitals from the business of illness management mainly, to include active strategies in health promotion, has been influenced by the WHO. Cullen (2002, p 41) describes a health promoting hospital as a WHO:

> . . . concept that strives to encourage hospitals to actively work towards being model healthy organizations. It adds another dimension to the already well established acute care service delivery provided by hospitals—that of taking action to promote the health of patients, staff and the community of which the hospital is a part.

The concept of health promoting hospitals is an exciting one for nurses, and involves a change from an almost exclusive focus on providing illness care in hospitals to one where the focus is on improving health. This means that people living with an acute or chronic illness need to be supported by nurses in their efforts to learn as much about their health problems as they can, and the treatments being offered to them. In this scenario, hospitals become much more than places where medical treatment is given and nursing care provided. In a health promoting hospital, health promotion is valued as a life process, and the recipients of health care are acknowledged as the key players in health promotion rather than the various health professionals (Cullen 2002). The active collaboration required to achieve health promotion of this kind reflects beliefs in partnership and proactivity in nursing that may come some distance in realising the WHO's definition of health, or the adjustments suggested to it by Saracci (1997) and McMurray (2003). These concepts of partnership are described in some detail in Chapter 12 of this text.

# Wellness

Health and health promotion are related to wellness and this section explores definitions of wellness, how it can be achieved as a way of life, and some research examining wellness factors. McMurray (2003, p 10) asserts that when 'people are healthy, they recognize the potential for higher levels of wellness'. She traces the origins of the definition of wellness to Dunn (1959, 1961), who emphasised dynamic relationships between people and their environments 'to maintain balance and purposeful direction' and the goal of 'living life at maximum potential and in harmony with the circumstances of one's life' (McMurray 2003, p 10).

## Case study . . . *continued*

During his teenage years, Andrew managed his asthma well. He was motivated by a desire to participate in as many sports as he could. He didn't feel like he was making up for the years of not being in sports when he was young, but recognised in himself a passion for sport itself. First he joined a swimming club. His parents were concerned that such activity might trigger asthma attacks, but Andrew convinced them to let him try. Over the years Andrew participated in basketball, tennis, and was a high school state representative in hockey. Andrew found that at this time in his life he was no longer experiencing the dreaded asthma attacks that had always been a feature of his illness. Well before his final year of high school, Andrew decided that he wanted to take up his passion for sports as a physical education teacher when he finished his school years.

Andrew's wellness improved because he was managing his asthma condition. This gave him the capacity to engage in sport, which then further enhanced his asthma management, and increased his confidence, sense of wellbeing and level of wellness.

Wellness is a broad and complex concept that has been described in the 'Wheel of Wellness' model (Sweeney & Witmer 1991, Witmer and Sweeney 1992). The original Wheel of Wellness proposed five life tasks interconnected and interrelated like spokes of a wheel, and these included spirituality, self-regulation, work, friendship and love. After research using an assessment instrument with 3000 people (The Wellness Evaluation of Lifestyle (WEL), Myers et al 2000), the original model was refined to divide the life task of 'work' into 'work and leisure' and to change the life task of 'self-regulation' into 'self-direction', the latter including twelve subtasks of sense of worth, sense of control, realistic beliefs, emotional awareness and coping, problem solving and creativity, sense of humour, nutrition, exercise, self-care, stress management, gender identity and cultural identity.

In spite of its complexities and challenges, the idea of wellness has been so well appropriated into the health care language and culture that a Distinguished Professor of Wellness and Gerontology in America suggests that the position of Surgeon General of the United States be converted to Wellness General of the United States (Haber 2002). He proposes changes to institutions and policies, including most notably for the general public, a tax on junk food, such as candy bars, cookies, cakes, pastries, ice cream, soft drink, corn chips and so on, that are the high fat, high sugar, high salt foods 'that constitute over 20% of Americans' calories' (p 73). His motivation in suggesting these reforms is 'to stimulate ideas and actions among policymakers, researchers, practitioners, educators, and students'. Interestingly, the general public is not included in the group to which his ideas are targeted, even though they would be affected directly by the changes he proposes to create family and community health. These well intentioned ideas carry overtones of the totalitarianism to which Saracci (1997) refers, in which it could be inferred that the general public will be required to embrace wellness, even if they choose to do otherwise.

Wellness is the subject of research projects that seek to explore its facilitation in a number of areas; for example, in disabilities (Putnam, Geenen & Powers 2003), physical activity (Bezner, Adams & Whistler 1999) and spiritual and psychological wellness (Adams & Bezner 2000).

Putnam et al (1999) used focus groups of two to ten participants for a total of 99 adults with long-term disabilities, to discuss with them how they define and conceptualise health and wellness and to explore with them their perceptions of barriers and facilitators in relation to living with disabilities. The participants defined health and wellness as (p 38):

- being able to function and do what they wanted to do;
- being independent or self-determining;
- having both a physical and emotional state of wellbeing, and
- an absence of pain.

Data also suggested that appropriate interventions are required at personal and community levels, within social and physical environments 'to facilitate greater levels of health and wellness among persons living with disability' (Putnam et al 1999, p 37).

Bezner et al (1999) surveyed a sample of 243 hospital employees using the Perceived Wellness Survey (Adams et al 1997), which is designed to assess wellness in physical, social, emotional, intellectual, psychological and spiritual dimensions. The results showed that higher scores for wellness were associated with participation in greater amounts of leisure time and moderate amounts of activity.

In a project involving 112 undergraduates enrolled in a health education class in Texas, USA, Adams & Bezner (2000) assessed the spiritual and psychological dimensions of wellness. The researchers found that 'an optimistic outlook and sense of coherence must be present for life purpose to enhance an overall sense of well-being' (Adams & Bezner 2000, p 165).

# Illness

Illness is perceived generally as the opposite to wellness and it is represented as something to be dreaded, avoided and treated, but the experiencing person may also see illness as something to be acknowledged, endured and valued for the life insights it offers. This section describes illness by differentiating it from disease, locating it on a continuum to wellness, and in exploring the rights and obligations of the sick role. Illness is also described from lay perspectives, patients' experiences, and social causes.

McMurray (2001, p 3) explains illness has been considered variously as 'ranging from disease, the presence of symptoms, or suffering, to deviance from normal expectations of good health'. However, unlike the objective state of disease, illness is also perceived as a 'subjective appraisal, in terms of how a person perceives or experiences ill health'. She gives the example of how two people may respond differently to the symptoms of the disease of diabetes and how they might interpret their disability uniquely, according to their inability to function at their usual level. She concludes that 'health, illness, disease, disability and wellness are therefore parts of the same process'.

Travis & Ryan (1981) devised a model for assessing a person's health level, by depicting a health–illness continuum from high-level wellness to severe illness. At the midpoint of the continuum are risk factors that may determine a person's propensity to be healthy or ill, such as genetic, environmental, social and cultural factors that are a compilation of all the inherent risks in being human and being involved in everyday life. For example, a person's cultural factors influencing their health or wellness may include dietary habits dictated by their respective social group's norms and traditions. It may be more common to detect higher rates of cardiac disease in cultural groups who eat high fat, high salt diets.

If a person becomes ill, how does one act differently from being well? The rights and obligations of a person who becomes sick have been documented in the well-known work of Talcott Parsons (1951), a sociologist, who described the sick role. Parsons claimed that sick people have the right to be exempt from their normal tasks and responsibilities, but that they need to want to get well to return again to the normal fabric of functioning society. He also suggested that sick people have the right not to be blamed for their illness, because they cannot be held responsible for it. However, they have an obligation to seek help from doctors and to cooperate with them in getting well as soon as possible. The underlying assumptions of the rights and obligations of the sick role are that the normal functioning of society relies on a healthy population and medical practice assists society and individuals to become and remain well, to assist in maintaining society and people in optimal biological, economic, psychological and social functioning.

How do lay people perceive illness? Schmidt & Frohling (2000) studied lay concepts of health and illness from a developmental perspective. They were interested in the nature of the concepts held by people of different age groups. Using a questionnaire, they explored with 99 children, and 48 mothers of the children, their perceptions of five diseases (cold, measles, heart infarction, cancer and AIDS). They found that many (p 230):

> . . . children and adolescents were able to define health positively (well-being) and not merely the absence of illness. The definition of illness in general was frequently composed of somatic symptoms and disorders, feeling poorly and things one would like to accomplish but can't.

## Case study ... *continued*

Andrew became a physical education teacher, highly thought of by his students and other teachers. Now, at 25 years of age, he was diagnosed with advanced bone cancer six months ago, news which he and his family found utterly devastating. Currently he is receiving palliative care from the local hospice team of nurses, doctors, and allied health workers. The team, mostly the nurses, have been visiting Andrew's home for three months, where he lives with his mother, father and teenage sister. Although Andrew had been living independently of his family for eight years, he has moved back home, because he knows he is dying and he wants to be with his family in his last weeks and days.

Andrew and his family have faced a very difficult time trying to come to terms with the nature of his illness. They have felt much supported by the nurses from the hospice, who have allowed them time to express their feelings and speak of their concerns. Always a close family, they have gained strength to confront this tragedy from the loving support they have received from many friends and also from the health professionals caring for Andrew.

In spite of his prognosis, Andrew expresses a certain love for life, as shown in his deep emotional bond to his family, his love of music, his enjoyment of visits from close friends, watching TV sports and his pleasure in smoking a joint daily.

Nurses need to be aware of lay perspectives of illness, to keep in touch with the general public, who are the consumers of health care services. For example, adequate explanations of illness, treatments and care regimes rely on having an understanding of the person's beginning knowledge, so being aware of lay perspectives can give nurses a good starting point for creating effective educational programs. For Andrew this might incorporate his passion for music as a relaxation technique and his deep bond to his family and love for his friends as his support network.

How do people experience illness? Patients' experiences of illness are receiving more attention and add to nurses' understanding of what it means to be ill. For example, Young-Mason (1997, p ix) documents 'autobiographical accounts of psychiatric and somatic illnesses' emphasising 'the implications of illness and spiritual distress and the ways in which individuals express their views of compassionate care'. The richness of patients' accounts is evidenced in the following excerpt from Allan McMurdy's (in Young-Mason (1997, p 9) account of living with muscular dystrophy:

> Muscular dystrophy and I are lifelong companions, and although I know our mortal enmity will some day be tested (and I will lose), we have maintained a relationship of wary coexistence. The disease and I were first introduced in the second grade when I was diagnosed, but we had been intimately connected from the moment my parents conceived me, their eldest son. As a genetic disorder, muscular dystrophy is as much a part of my identity as my eye color, my height, or my resemblance to my parents. It was never an invader:

the disease and I have fought for control over territory to which we both felt entitled.

Other stories within the collection (Young-Mason 1997) are as told by the mother of Raoul, a 27-year-old man with cerebral palsy (pp 18–33), and of Gertrude, aged 11, with a long medical history because of being born prematurely with multiple systems abnormality (pp 35–39). Even though their experiences of illness have included many challenges and struggles, they are able to celebrate their small daily triumphs and offer words of insightful wisdom to health care professionals. For example, Raoul's mother concluded her account of 27 years of trying to help and educate her son, by writing:

> Does Raoul know he is missing out on so much of life's experience? Is he aware of his difference? Sometimes I think so, but I'll probably never know for sure. Raoul remains innocent and is therefore one of the more vulnerable members of our society. I continue to worry for him. How will he cope with life when I am no longer here for him? But then I remember how many people have already been touched by Raoul . . . I'm left with some of my dearest memories, like putting Raoul to bed, closing the door, and hearing 'Mom?' 'Yes, Raoul.' 'What if the bus doesn't come?' 'Don't worry, it will come in the morning. Go to sleep.' 'Mom?' 'Don't worry, I love you.'

Experiences of illness are central to improving health care. The accounts of people experiencing illness offer nurses deep insights into how it is to be ill and how it is to care for someone you love who is ill. When illness becomes a lifetime experience, it becomes assimilated into daily life and integrates into ordinary human activities. In becoming assimilated, illness loses some of its biomedical objectivity as it infuses into the uncomplicated reality of activities such as unplugging the kitchen sink, peeling the vegetables for dinner and putting out the garbage. The ordinary, everyday lives of people and how they manage illness are instructive for nurses who may espouse to offer healing to patients through holistic caring practices. Experiences of illness are a cornerstone of this text, and you will find that many other chapters offer more insights into what it is like to be ill.

Lay and professional people inhabit the social world and they influence, and are in turn influenced by, the social causes of illness. Teschendorff (2001, p 48) contends that even though there are multi-causal determinants of health and illness, such as specific environmental and individual factors, that health care providers focus on these factors and neglect 'broader environmental, political and socioeconomic factors'. She exemplifies this point by listing the disadvantages faced by 'the underprivileged in society' such as 'social dislocation, unemployment, disempowerment and poverty'. These disadvantages are discussed in depth in Chapter 3.

# Healing

The holistic caring practices of nurses may result in healing. It is important to consider what is meant by the word healing in this sense, as it is often confused with curing. Healing does not necessarily involve curing, although some or total cure may be evident in the healing process. The distinction between healing and curing is that healing is felt as a relative state of being, while curing is demonstrated by objective evidence; for example, in surgical wound healing. In contrast, emotional wounds may have no hope or evidence of cure by treatments and procedures; rather they may require healing of a different nature. The kind of healing that is mediated through therapeutic relationships is redefined 'as moments in which beneficial differences are perceived' (Taylor 1995, p 100) and as when 'one knows that progress has been made on a forward path, that moves one closer to a fuller sense of self, whether it be towards improved health or towards a peaceful death' (p 105). Andrew's nurses realised that there was no hope of a cure for him. He was going to die of his cancer. However, their actions in caring for him emotionally as well as physically were healing because he was able to speak of his feelings and feel understood. He found this took an enormous burden from him.

While healing may seem like difficult work, it may mean no more than being attentive to the quality of intrapersonal and interpersonal relationships and making sense of, and learning from, the constant array of life's joys and woes. For example, it simply requires taking notice of and practising seemingly small things, such as activities that have the potential to transmit authentic qualities of love, caring, compassion, kindness, forgiveness, patience, respect, trust and hope.

How do we know that healing has occurred? Dossey et al (2000, p 42) warn that:

> It is one thing to evaluate whether the signs and symptoms of a disease are still present. It is quite another to determine if there has been a shift at any level of this person's body–mind–spirit.

The authors suggest that the answer to the conundrum of whether healing is happening, is by the 'subjective knowing of the patient and nurse' (Dossey et al 2000, p 42), when both know that something special has happened, even though there 'may be no words, no description, just knowing'. They explain that 'neither may be able to name what the healing was, what shifted, but they trust that it is real' (p 43). Often the deepest meanings cannot be conveyed, rather they are experienced, recognised and left to be—knowing that they have made a difference. For example, when a person feels acknowledged, it may be through the most ordinary behaviours, such as a nod, smile, or a well-placed word. The acknowledgment in turn creates a healing effect, such as the loss of anxiety or 'heartache'. The possibility that healing is a process of self-awareness and emergence and that it is relevant to health care, is subsumed within the wider parameters of holism and holistic practice.

# Holism

It is accepted generally that the person who first coined the term 'holism' was Jan Smuts (1926) who was then the President of South Africa. In referring to the States of South Africa, he described entities and systems as unified wholes with dynamic interdependence of their parts and suggested that wholes be understood in their totality as greater than the sum of their parts. For Smuts (1926, p v) holism was 'the principle which makes for the origin and progress of wholes in the universe'. Cmich (1984) explained four principles of holism as: the principle is that entities and systems in the universe are unified wholes; the parts of the whole are dynamically inter-dependent and interrelated; a whole cannot be understood isolated from its parts; and the whole is greater than the sum of its parts.

## Case study . . . *continued*

Increasingly, Andrew's pain is becoming non-responsive to large doses of narcotic analgesics. He is also very uncomfortable from a large bedsore in his sacral area, which formed in spite of the nurses' best attempts to prevent it by changes of position and a modified bed mattress to relieve pressure. Andrew is a shy man, who does not like the health team peering at his sacrum, although he cooperates with the dressing changes and pressure relief measures.

Holism in health care developed as a reaction to reductionist health care, reflected in the care of body parts, like bits of a machine needing technology and clinical procedures to fix malfunctions. This scientific model developed from reductionism was embraced by medicine, because it provided a framework for answering questions about the complexity of the human body, and biomedical science has made many advances because of it. Chapter 8 includes a useful discussion about the biomedical model, and how it has affected the care of the ill.

However, when the biomedical model took objective information about the structure and function of the human body, and subsequently deperson-alised humans who are ill, there was a need to return to holistic approaches to people and their health care. Based on the assumption that people are greater than the sum of their parts, holistic health takes into account the dynamic nature of the wholeness of people and relies on their potential as humans to bring about the best outcomes for themselves and their environ-ments. For example, Andrew's expertise in asthma management and familiarity with hospitals and nurses could be utilised by nurses to assist him with the discomfort he experiences during dressing changes, through explanation and involving him in decisions about his treatment.

As one of the catch-cries of the contemporary era, much has been written about holism in relation to health (Benner 1984, Brennan 1987, 1993, Fergusson 1976, Hetzel 1991, Janiger & Goldberg 1993, Keegan 1994, Rogers 1969, Thompson 1994) and the concept has been subjected to a thorough critique (Beyerstein 1997, Bohm 1980, Bruni 1989, Green 1997, Kermode &

## Living with Illness

Brown 1995, Kramer 1990, Madjar 1987, Owen 1995, Popper 1974, Smith 1988, Sobel 1979, Williams 1988). Holism has been applied in medicine (Newell 2000, Scott 1999) and nursing (Buckley 2002, Long & Baxter 2001, Taylor 2002) and even though it has limitations in its interpretation and application, it nevertheless remains the ideal for nurses' practice in their intention to view people as dynamic, whole beings deserving of high quality body–mind–spirit care.

Nurses try to practice in such a way as to maintain the integrity of the whole person, in the face of multiple losses associated with illness and/or in eventual deterioration towards death. Insight into a patient's attempt to keep her body–mind–spirit intact and connected while facing death was recorded eloquently by Bolletino (2000, p 57) in 'an experiential case for holism'. The author summarised the disintegration of self of Anna Cassirer Applebaum, a psychotherapist, who:

> . . . died on May 28, 1998, six days before her ninetieth birthday. Technically, the cause of her death was congestive heart failure. Actually, she died from erosion. Everything except her fine mind wore out and broke down. During the last few months of her life she became interested in what she noticed about her physical deterioration and its effects. She realised that her experiences were different from accepted assumptions about aging and physical loss, and decided to write a paper. So she became a 'participant observer', working to examine her own decline . . . Anna's observations constituted a definite case for holism. They leave no doubt that we human beings are organic wholes, no part or function of which can be lost without serious distortion and damage to our wholeness and sense of identity. Her observations also show that our concrete experience of the world around us is inseparable from our experience of our selves.

In eroding towards death, Anna was losing her eyesight and her sense of touch, taste, smell and, worst of all, her hearing, because she had a lifelong love of music. In observing her disintegrating self, Anna came to the conclusion that (p 71):

> . . . now I have lost the design, the world becomes totally senseless, and in a sensless world, you realy get chaotic. The whole organisation falls apart, and all that God created out of chaos goes back to chaos.

This eloquent summation of health as wholeness and deterioration as erosion of parts creates the possibility that in falling apart and becoming chaotic, maybe death reintegrates the human spirit in absolute oneness. Such a hope cannot be considered too fanciful if we truly believe that holism includes a spiritual dimension.

# Holistic nursing and healing partnerships

Holistic nursing is (Taylor 2002, p 64):

> . . . a comprehensive way of being, knowing and doing in the delivery of knowledgeable, skilful and human centered nursing care, which relates to people as greater than the sum of their parts.

This definition emphasises the integration of a nurse's knowledge, skills and humanity in the intention of providing care that reflects, as far as humanly possible, the intention to relate to the totality of the patient's body–mind–spirit. One of the reasons why holism is critiqued is that it is an ideal (Bruni 1989, Madjar 1987, Owen 1995), which is very difficult to attain in the busyness of everyday practice, so it is not surprising that some nurses remain objective yet polite, doing their work safely, systematically and on time, with little or no intention to practise holistically.

When nurses choose to work in clinical and fragmented ways, devoid of the therapeutic use of self through authentic interpersonal connection, and without consideration of the multidimensional nature of patients' contexts, they are not practising holistically (Taylor 2002, p 64).

If nurses remain detached and objective in professional interpersonal relationships, it is unlikely that they will create healing partnerships with patients. For example, decades ago Jourard (1971) criticised the tendency of people to hide away behind masks in their daily interactions. He claimed that we (pp vii–viii):

> . . . camouflage our true being before others to protect ourselves against criticism and rejection. This protection comes at a steep price. When we are not truly known by the other people in our lives, we are misunderstood. When we are misunderstood, especially by family and friends, we join the 'lonely crowd'. Worse, when we succeed in hiding our being from others, we tend lose touch with our real selves. This loss of self contributes to illness in its myriad forms.

Jourard was especially critical of nurses of that time, although he added 'with a little imagination on the reader's part' that what he had to say could relate also to 'physicians, teachers, clergymen (sic), dentists, lawyers, counsellors and psychotherapists—anyone working in a "helping" profession' (p 177). In speaking of the 'bedside manner', Jourard listed the inauthentic behaviours of nurses that maintain their distance between, and superiority over, patients in their care. He said that nurses adopt rigid behaviours and wear 'character armor' to protect them against the potential hurts in their practice. He advocated that all health care professionals strive to work from a 'transparent self', which is open to other people and true to oneself. Such suggestions for communication in health care systems of the early 1970s were indeed radical and are still relevant today.

To be able to take off the mask of detachment and create authenticity within the patient–carer relationship requires some 'emotional labour' (Hochschild 1979, 1983) on the part of the health professional. Hochschild (1983) considered that employees who had person-to-person contact with the general public were under an obligation from their employers to exercise some control in managing their emotions for the good of the organisation. This means that 'emotional labourers' have prescribed and defined behaviours that keep the employers and the consumers happy with the service of the organisation. Hochschild (1983) added that managing one's emotions requires active deep acting when employees work hard to manage emotions, and passive deep acting, when the employees spontaneously feel what they are required to feel. Since Hochschild's foundational work, there have been many critiques (Conrad & Witte 1994, Wharton & Erikson 1993) and research projects (Henderson 2001, Kruml & Geddes 2000, Staden 1998) relating to emotional labour, and it provides a useful concept for considering the degree of authenticity that is possible and therapeutic in public work, such as nursing.

In moving from active deep acting (expressing feigned emotions) to passive deep acting (expressing true emotions), nurses may choose to attempt to create therapeutic relationships with patients based on mutuality, trust and reciprocity (Muetzel 1988). Emotions can become authentic, from a basis of respectful caring, thus making them potentially therapeutic.

## Case study . . . *continued*

Kate was one of the nurses providing home-based hospice care to Andrew and his family. Over the weeks she had been working with Andrew and his family, she had come to deeply respect and care for them, and felt saddened by what was happening for them. One day, whilst attending to Andrew's physical needs, Kate broke down and started to cry. She was horrified, because she was there to help not make the situation even more unbearable. At Andrew's funeral, to her surprise, his father in his eulogy said that Andrew had spoken of that incident afterwards, saying that he felt a renewal of strength and energy when he realised how much Kate cared.

According to the Australian Oxford Dictionary, the word therapeutic is derived from the Greek *therapeutikos*, meaning 'to wait on, cure' and the word therapist is derived from the Greek *therapeia*, meaning 'healing' (Moore 1999). In health care, therapeutics has moved from a disease-curing meaning relating mainly in doctors, to healing through caring facilitated by the emotional work of nurses, social workers, occupational therapists and other health professionals. All health care professionals can choose to use their presence to give therapeutic care, thereby forming healing partnerships with patients.

Nurses recognise the therapeutic value of the nurse–patient relationship in collaboration and partnership in health care (Downie et al 2001, Gassner et al 1999, Keatinge et al 2002, McQueen 2000) and are also aware of its potential (Spitzer 2002, Weir 2001). The healing partnership lies in the ability to connect with clients, based on the nature and quality of human relationships. Taylor (1994, 2000) suggests one way to conceptualise this relationship is through 'ordinariness', which is the nature of being human. She claims that nurses and patients share a common sense of humanity. Within the context of caring, patients attune themselves with nurses, because of their sense of affinity as humans. At the same time, patients acknowledge nurses' knowledge and skills and allow themselves to be supported by their professional qualities and activities. Shared humanity can be applied anywhere humans interact. Ordinariness is common to all humans, therefore, it presents some possibilities for all health care professionals who are keen to create healing partnerships with patients.

In a public health context, healing partnerships also refer to community and consumer participation in health (Johnson 2001, p 25). Increasingly, the public is being encouraged to voice their needs and concerns to provide safety and quality in health care. Johnson (2001, p 25) suggests that consumers' participation can be encouraged through education and support, so they can participate actively 'in decision-making in individual care processes, health services and the broader health system'. Although consumer partnerships in this context may appear to differ from the healing partnerships attained through interpersonal connection, it can also be inferred that only those consumers who are empowered through education, trust, respect and communication (Keatinge et al 2002), will be likely to want to be involved in consumer participation in health processes and policies.

## Summary

This chapter introduced the concepts of health, wellness, illness, healing and holism, holistic nursing, 'emotional labour' and therapeutic relationships. These ideas are foundational to understanding the psychosocial challenges in living with illness. Nurses interact daily with people to attain and maintain health and wellness. Understanding the experience of illness from lay and patients' viewpoints leads to a deeper appreciation of the human body–mind–spirit and potentiates the likelihood that holistic health care will be espoused and enacted in work settings. Therapeutic relationships between patients and professional health carers facilitate healing and partnership and they are integral to authentic interpersonal interactions in health care settings.

## Tutorial questions

1. What definition of health do you prefer, and why?
2. How is health different from wellness?
3. How is healing different from curing?
4. What are the perceived benefits of holistic nursing?
5. What is meant by healing partnerships?

**Questions 6–9 relate to the case study:**

6. In what ways might it be perceived that Andrew is healthy, well and/or ill when he was child and an adult?
7. Is healthy dying possible?

8.  If the health team are to care for Andrew holistically, what dimensions of his illness experience do they need to assess?
9.  Is a one-to-one therapeutic relationship possible with Andrew if a particular member of the health team objects to Andrew smoking dope?

# References

Adams T, Bezner J 2000 Conceptualization and measurement of the spiritual and psychological dimensions of wellness in a college population. *Journal of American College Health* 48(4):165–174

Adams TA, Bezner JB, Steinhardt MA 1997 The conceptualization and management of wellness: Integrating balance across and within dimensions. *American Journal of Health Promotion* 11(3):208–218

Benner P 1984 *From Novice to Expert: Excellence and Power in Clinical Nursing Practice.* Addison-Wesley, Menlo Park

Beyerstein B 1997 Why bogus therapies seem to work. *Skeptical Inquirer* September/October 21(5):29–34

Bezner J, Adams T, Whistler L 1999 The relationship between physical activity and indicators of perceived wellness. *American Journal of Health Studies* 15(3):130–138

Bohm D 1980 *Wholeness and the Implicate Order.* Routledge and Kegan Paul, London

Bolletino R 2000 Observations on the disintegration of the self: An experiential case for holism. *Advances in Mind-Body Medicine* 16(1):57–71

Brennan BA 1987 *Light Emerging: The Journey of Personal Healing.* Bantam Books, New York

Brennan BA 1993 *Hands of Light: A Guide to Healing Through the Human Energy Field.* Bantam Books, Toronto

Bright MA 2002 *Holistic Health and Healing.* FA Davis Co, Philadelphia

Bruni N 1989 Holism: A radical nursing perspective, paper presented to National Nursing Theory Conference South Australian College of Advanced Education in Koch T ed, *Theory and practice; An evolving relationship*, The School of Nursing Studies Sturt

Buckley J 2002 Holism and a health-promoting approach to palliative care. *International Journal of Palliative Care* 8(10):505–508

Cmich DE 1984 Theoretical perspectives on holistic health. *Journal of School Health* 2:30–32

Conrad C, Witte K 1994 Is emotional expression repression oppression? Myths of organization affective regulation. In: Deetz S (ed) *Communication Yearbook.* Sage, California

Cullen A 2002 *Health promotion in the changing face of the hospital landscape.* Collegian 9(1):41–42

Dossey B, Keegan L, Guzzetta C 2000 *Holistic Nursing: A Handbook for Practice*, 3rd edn. Aspen, Gaithersburg

Downie J, Orb A, Wynaden D, McGowan S, Seeman Z, Ogilvie S 2001 A practice-research model for collaborative partnership. *Collegian* 8(4):27–32

Dunn H 1959 High-level wellness for man and society. *American Journal of Public Health* 49:789. In McMurray A 2003, Community Health and Wellness: A Sociological Approach, 2nd edn. Mosby, Sydney

## 2: Health, Wellness, Illness, Healing and Holism, and Nursing

Dunn H 1961 What high-level wellness means, Health Values 1:9. In: Mc Murray A, 2003 *Community Health and Wellness: A Sociological Approach*, 2nd edn. Mosby, Sydney

Ferguson M C 1976 Nursing at the crossroads: Which way to turn? A look at the model of nurse practitioner, *Journal of Advanced Nursing* 1(3):237–242

Gassner L-A, Wotton K, Clare J, Hofmeyer A, Buckman J 1999 Theory meets practice—Evaluation of a model of collaboration: academic and clinical partnership in the development and implementation of undergraduate teaching. *Collegian*, 6(3):14–21

Green S 1997 Pseudoscience in alternative medicine. *Skeptical Inquirer,* September/October, 21(5):1–5

Haber D 2002 Wellness general of the United States: A creative approach to promote family and community health. *Family Community Health* 25(3):71–82

Henderson A 2001 Emotional labor and nursing: An under-appreciated aspect of caring work. *Nursing Inquiry* 8(2):130–139

Hetzel R 1991 *The New Physician: Tapping the Potential for True Health*. Houghton Mifflin Australia, Victoria

Hochschild A 1979 Emotion work, feeling roles, and social structure. *American Journal of Sociology* 85:551–575

Hochschild A 1983 *The Managed Heart: Commmercialization of Human Feeling*. University of California Press, Berkeley

Janiger O, Goldberg P 1993 *A Different Kind of Healing: Doctors Speak Candidly About Their Successes with Alternative Medicine*. Putnam Books, New York

Johnson A 2001 An outline of consumer participation in health. *Collegian* 8(2):25–27

Jourard SM 1971 *The Transparent Self*. D Van Nostrand Company, New York

Keatinge D, Bellchambers H, Bujack E, Cholowski K, Conway J, Neal P 2002 Communication: Principal barrier to nurse–consumer partnerships. *International Journal of Nursing Practice* 8(1):16–22

Keegan L 1994 *The Nurse as Healer*. Delmar Publishers, Albany

Kermode S, Brown C 1995 Where have all the flowers gone: Nursing's escape from the radical critique. *Contemporary Nurse* 4(1):8–15

Kramer MK 1990 Holistic nursing: Implications for knowledge development and utilisation. In: N Chaska (ed) *The Nursing Profession: Turning Points*. CV Mosby, St Louis, pp. 245–54

Kruml S, Geddes D 2000 Exploring the dimensions of emotional labor: The heart of Hochschild's work. *Management Communication Quarterly* 14(1):8–49

Long A, Baxter R 2001 Functionalism and holism: Community nurses' perceptions of health. *Journal of Clinical Nursing* 10(3):320–330

Madjar I 1987 *Wholistic nursing: Challenges options choices*, Paper presented at the Challenges Options Choices International Conference New Zealand Nurses Association Rotorua, pp 1–12

McMurray A 2001 Health and Wellness. In: Crisp J and Taylor C (eds), 2001 *Potter and Perry's Fundamentals of Nursing*. Mosby, Sydney, pp 1–19

McMurray A 2003 *Community Health and Wellness: A Sociological Approach*, 2nd edn. Mosby, Sydney

McQueen A 2000 Nurse–patient relationships and partnership in hospital care. *Journal of Clinical Nursing* 9(5):723–731

Meutzel PA 1988 Therapeutic nursing. In: A Pearson (ed), *Primary Nursing*. Croom Helm, London

Moore B (ed), 1999 *Australian Oxford Dictionary*, Oxford University Press, Oxford

Myers J, Sweeney T, Witmer J 2000 The wheel of wellness counseling for wellness: A holistic model for treatment planning. *Journal of Counseling and Development* 78(3):251–267

Newell C 2000 Biomedicine, genetics and disability: Reflections on nursing and a philosophy of holism. *Nursing Ethics* 7(3):227–237

Owen MJ 1995 Challenges to caring: Nurses' interpretation of holism. *The Australian Journal of Holistic Nursing* 2(2):4–14

Parsons T 1951 Illness and the role of the Physician: A sociological perspective. *American Journal of Orthopsychiatry* 21:452–466

Popper KD 1974 *The Open Society and its Enemies:* Volume 2: Hegel and Marx. Routledge and Kegan Paul, London

Putnam M, Geenen S, Powers L 2003 Health and wellness: people with disabilities discuss barriers and facilitators to well being. *Journal of Rehabilitation* 69(1):37–45

Rogers M 1969 *Introduction to the Theoretical Basis of Nursing*. Davis, New York

Saracci R 1997 The World Health Organization needs to reconsider its definition of health. *British Medical Journal* 314(7091):1409–1411

Schmidt L, Frohling H 2000 Lay concepts of health and illness from a developmental perspective. *Psychology and Health* 15(2):229–239

Scott A 1999 Paradoxes of holism: Some problems in developing an anti-oppressive medical practice. *Health* 3(2):131–149

Smith MJ 1988 Perspectives on wholeness: The lens makes a difference. *Nursing Science Quarterly* 1(3):94–95

Smith M 2002 Health, healing, and the myth of the hero journey. *Advances in Nursing Science* 24(4):1–13

Smuts JC 1926, Holism and Evolution. MacMillan, New York

Sobel DS 1979 *Ways of Health: Holistic Approaches to Ancient and Contemporary Medicine*. Harcourt Brace Jovanovich, New York

Spitzer O 2002 The role of the therapeutic relationship. *Diversity* 2(7):17–23

Staden H 1998 Alertness to the needs of others: A study of the emotional labour of caring. *Journal of Advanced Nursing* 27(1):147–156

Sweeney T, Witmer J 1991 Beyond social interest: Striving toward optimal health and wellness. *Individual Psychology* 47:527–540

Taylor B 2002 Becoming a reflective nurse or midwife: using complementary therapies while practising holistically. *Complementary Therapies in Nursing and Midwifery* 8(4):62–68

Taylor BJ 1994 *Being Human: Ordinariness in Nursing*. Churchill Livingstone, Melbourne

Taylor B 1995 Nursing as healing work. *Contemporary Nurse.* 4(3):100–106

Taylor B 2000 *Being Human: Ordinariness in Nursing* (Adapted and reprinted). Southern Cross University Press, Lismore

Teschendorff J 2001 Does holistic medicine ignore the social causes of illness? *Diversity* 2(4):46–51

Thompson I 2002 Mental health and spiritual care. *Nursing Standard* 17(9):33–39

Thompson P 1994 *Finding Your Own Spiritual Path: An Everyday Guidebook*. Hazelton, Minnesota

Travis JW, Ryan RS 1981 *Wellness Workbook*. Ten Speed Press, California

Warrawee'a KL-D 2000 Neetsa: An Aboriginal perspective on holistic health. *Diversity* 2(2):2–9

Weir M 2001 The ten commandments of professional practice. *Journal of Traditional-Medicine Society* 7(1):9–13

Wharton A, Erikson R 1993 Managing emotion on the job and at home: Understanding the consequences of multiple emotional roles. *Academy of Management Review* 18:457–486

Williams K 1988 World view and the facilitation of wholeness. *Holistic Nursing Practice* 2(3):1–8

Witmer JM, Sweeney TJ 1992 A holistic model of wellness and prevention over the life span. *Journal of Counseling and Development* 71:140–148.

World Health Organization (WHO) 1974 Basic Documents 36thed. WHO, Geneva

Young-Mason J 1997 *The Patient's Voice: Experiences of Illness*. FA Davis Company, Philadelphia

# Chapter 3

## Class, Poverty and Illness: Intersecting Links

*Jan Horsfall*

**This chapter:**

- outlines upstream, midstream and downstream contributions to chronic illness, specifically heart disease;
- explores the meaning of socially structured inequality;
- defines and explains class and poverty;
- defines mortality, years of life lost, and morbidity; and
- discusses some nursing strategies to offset socially structured health inequalities.

This chapter discusses the concepts of class, socioeconomic status and poverty. It explains their relationship to long-term illness using Turrell and Mathers' (2000) model, which outlines three levels of factors that contribute to many long-term illnesses. The relationship between class and mortality rates, years of life lost and morbidity rates are also explained by drawing on Australian and overseas research. The chapter will emphasise that people with lower socioeconomic status in Australia are more likely to die early of coronary heart disease (CHD), therefore a case study of CHD will be used in this chapter. When the medical symptoms of CHD are explored in this way, it should become clear to you that a person's area of residence, education level and income underpin their stress at work, poor diet, and decreased access to prevention services and early treatment. This understanding should help you formulate some strategies to lessen the burden of CHD. Chris's story about his heart attack begins the chapter.

## Case study

Chris is shorter than the male average, has a stocky build with much of his excess weight carried in front and above the waist. Chris began cigarette smoking at 14, smoked 20 a day from age 18, and smoked at least 40 cigarettes a day from age

27, rising to 80 per day. His father died of a heart attack at the age of 35, when Chris was in primary school. Chris works hard at his job and went through a period when he had many demands made on him from both above and below. He says that he has high expectations of himself and others and tends to take on a lot of responsibility.

The last five years of his life have been a medical nightmare. Chris was diagnosed with chronic fatigue syndrome five years ago, which required nine months off work. He was then diagnosed with non-insulin dependent diabetes 18 months ago after having diabetic symptoms for a year beforehand. Neither of these diagnoses prompted him to take any actions to improve his basic health. His diabetes is treated with medication. Exercise was not part of his lifestyle at this time, and he had not had his cholesterol tested. When I asked him how he was able to ignore the risks to his health he said he was 'comfortable in my addictions, and anyhow I just didn't believe that I would have a heart attack'.

Six months ago, at the age of 50, he did have a heart attack. Chris underwent coronary bypass surgery after his heart attack and was advised to give up smoking. He used nicotine patches for three weeks and had completely stopped smoking three months later. Chris participated in a cardiac rehabilitation program (physical and education) and returns every two weeks to reinforce/maintain his efforts. Now he walks regularly; is eating more fruit and vegetables; has cut down on sweet and refined carbohydrate-based foods and consequently lost weight. Chris' wife and children have been worried about his health and are very supportive of his efforts to change his health-related behaviours. His employer is understanding and flexible and, after three months off work, he now works 18 hours a week, and if he works more it is on his own initiative. Chris understands that his coronary heart disease is a chronic condition, and that its management will require his life-long commitment.

## Explanatory model for coronary heart disease

Turrell and Mathers (2000) outline a model of *upstream* (closer to the source of the problem), *midstream* and *downstream* factors that determine whether people like Chris will develop heart disease. These risk factors are synergistic; that is, the combinations of factors interact to produce a compounding effect rather than being additive (Higginbotham et al 2001, p 94). Throughout this chapter, you should come to realise how interrelated all of these factors are, and that Chris' health problems are likely to have resulted from a combination of factors from all three levels of this model rather than one specific element.

## Upstream factors

Upstream, or macrosocial factors, include economic, political, and tax policies as well as employment status, education, income, and area of residence. For example, upstream factors influencing the development of Chris' health problems might also include the poverty he experienced in early childhood, especially after his father died. Worldwide, poverty is a serious threat to the health of several billion people (Horton 2003, p 713), so it is worthwhile discussing in some detail here.

Poverty is defined as 'as a state of deprivation, a situation where one's standard of living has fallen below some acceptable minimal level' (Harding, Lloyd & Greenwell 2002, p 2). Social scientists who research poverty have focused on relative poverty where the after-tax income of a family is lower in comparison to the average income for that size family in a specific nation at that time. Up to 17.5% of Australians live in financial hardship and, not surprisingly, more than half of unemployed people live in poverty (Harding et al 2002). Their vulnerability is also increasing, reflecting the slower increase in unemployment benefits during the late 1990s in comparison to average wages (Harding et al 2002).

Traditionally, women constituted the biggest group of poor people. Australia's first and only formal inquiry into poverty in the early 1970s found that women and children were over-represented amongst the poor (George & Davis 1998). People living in sole parent families continue to face the highest risk of poverty of all family types. Twenty-two per cent of sole parent families lived in poverty in Australia in 2000 (Harding et al 2002). Given that his father died prematurely, Chris was living as a child and teenager in a female-headed sole parent family during the 1960s. For many decades, and until very recently, there was very little medical research into CHD in women. One terrible consequence of this is that, at present, women living in poverty are 124 times more likely to die from CHD than wealthier women (Higgin-botham et al 2001). Women's symptoms can differ from men's, they receive less thorough investigations, are likely to be diagnosed later, be treated less aggressively in cardiac emergencies, have less family support during rehabil-itation, and return to work sooner (Gorman 2003).

Children remain the age group most vulnerable to poverty, rising to 15% of Australian children in 2000 (Harding et al 2002). This is disconcerting, given that poorer adult health is greatest among those who had childhood disadvantage similar to that experienced by Chris. Children from poorer families are more likely to be underweight at birth; become developmentally delayed; experience higher rates of pedestrian accidents; and have long-term health problems (Turrell & Mathers 2000). Thus, disease risk accumulates over a lifetime and the worst health accrues to those with the highest levels of economic and social adversity.

The economic and social adversity that Chris experienced as a child can be the result of inequalities between social groups, which are often explained in terms of class. Social class is one of those in-built differences between groups of people in a given society that is commonly unnoticed, or accepted as 'the way things are' and therefore not questioned. Such fundamental inequalities relate to what cannot be chosen. For example, in general neither we, nor our parents, can choose the income level of our parents, our gender, race, or class. These are circumstances into which we are born.

Class is defined as a 'position within a system of structured inequality based on the unequal distribution of power, wealth [and] income . . .' (Germov 2002, p 68). In a western capitalist country like Australia, class refers to groups of people on the basis of economic ownership and political power. The upper class owns economic resources, such as raw materials, technology and businesses. It includes senior executives and managers who have indisputable control over workers and access to profits through very high incomes and significant share holdings. Power and wealth remain concentrated within the upper class (Giddens 2001). The working class is made up of unskilled or semi-skilled workers who work in factories, offices and other settings. The middle class is differentiated from the working class by a combination of higher skill level, better working conditions and less vulnerability to market forces (predictable or unpredictable) that create unemployment and limited re-training opportunities. According to this three-stage explanation of class, 9% of Australians belong to the upper class; 47% to the middle class; and 44% to the working class (Germov 2002).

The term socioeconomic status (SES) is based on a less critical view of structured inequalities in comparison to the class model. SES is defined as the hierarchical ranking of people according to income, occupation, level of education and area of residence, and then grouping them into high, medium, and low SES groups.

## Midstream factors

Midstream or microsocial determinants of health include psychosocial factors like the individual's control of stress, life circumstances, demand strain at work and home, social support, self-esteem and coping skills. Health behaviours such as diet, cigarette smoking, alcohol and physical activity are also midstream factors. Chris has several of the known midstream risk factors for developing heart disease, including cigarette smoking and high body mass index. Midstream factors, such as ignoring healthy lifestyle information, clearly played their part in increasing his risk of developing CHD over many decades.

Studies have shown that people like Chris, who had little control over his work, are at greater risk for heart disease, musculoskeletal problems and mental disorders such as depression (Marmot 2000). In fact, some research shows that job strain more than doubles the death rate from CHD (Kivimaki et al 2002). Job strain relates to a combination of work demands, such as high levels of responsibility, task difficulty and mental load; along with low job control as evidenced by lack of decision making autonomy and skill discretion. These two work-related factors—effort reward imbalance and job strain—are clearly related to class. Working class people employed as unskilled or semi-skilled labour will experience effort–reward imbalance in high demand jobs, involving work pace, high levels of supervision, and long hours (Higginbotham et al 2001). Skilled working class and middle class employees like Chris will experience job strain in positions with high respon-sibility and low levels of policy and managerial power and autonomy, even though their education or training prepare them for expert autonomous decision-making. So although he came from a lower class family, Chris now considers himself to be middle class—and he certainly is not poor or uneducated. However, he has not been in control of his work circumstances and has experienced considerable pressure to produce results from both employers and clients—which has contributed directly to his chronic illness.

## Downstream factors

Downstream determinants of health are non-modifiable and include gender, age, genetic inheritance; as well as endocrine or immunological outcomes such as hypertension, fibrin production, excessive blood lipid levels, glucose intolerance and high body mass index (Turrell 2002, Turrell & Mathers 2000). Chris's family history indicates that he may have a predisposition to these factors, as do his high blood pressure and raised cholesterol levels. Chris's gender is also included in the non-modifiable risk category—before the age of 50, men are more likely to develop CHD than women.

Clearly, mid- and upstream factors have played a part in Chris' disease process and have exacerbated the risks related to the downstream factors he has little control over. For example, a downstream factor such as blood pressure increases in response to midstream factors such as obesity, high alcohol consumption, and the over-use of salt. Smoking more than doubles the incidence of CHD (Higginbotham et al 2001). Similarly, raised cholesterol is a by-product of a diet high in saturated fat, excessive alcohol intake and cigarette smoking, as well as insufficient exercise and being overweight. It could be that factors such as the class and income of his family of origin laid the foundations for midstream negative health-related behaviours. Another midstream factor is proposed by Heading (1996) who has identified one group of people as health promotion 'resisters' (cited in Higginbotham et al 2001). Resisters are mostly men who know the facts about lifestyle and heart attack risk, but who choose not to initiate positive changes in eating, smoking or exercise. Chris could be described as a 'resister'. Downstream factors of heredity and ageing come into play against this general background of an unhealthy lifestyle and resistance to a healthy one.

Turrell and Mather's (2000) model is a useful way to demonstrate that the biological factors that contribute to the risk of disease can occur because of a range of psychosocial factors, including a person's health-related behaviours. These factors are, in turn, influenced by economic, environmental and social stressors, having a cumulative effect upon a person's health. It has been recognised for some time that justice and equity of access to health services should be a key principle in public health that may address mid- and upstream factors (Drevdahl et al 2001, p 22). It is also well known, however, that injustices and inequity of access to health services contribute to poorer health outcomes for poorer people. These class-based factors must be taken into account by policy makers, including nurses, so that health policy and programs identify effective strategies to prevent CHD and other long-term illnesses in all sectors of our society. One way of determining equitable distribution of health resources is to use standard measures of health and illness inequalities. These are discussed in the following section.

# Measuring health and illness inequalities

There is a class gradient for morbidity (illness rates) and mortality (death rates) in our society. That is, the lower a person's class position, the greater the rate of illness and earlier death (Sainsbury & Harris 2001). This has been known for more than a century. In the first half of the twentieth century, western nations institutionalised clean water and efficient sewage disposal, established welfare systems, broadened the education base, and enabled basic health care to be accessed by the majority of the population. The gap between the death rates of the rich and poor then decreased for a few decades. In the second half of the twentieth century, such countries focused more on expanding production, market creation and increased domestic consumption. Therefore, the gap between rich and poor has increased since the 1970s—the time when Chris was cementing many of his health care behaviours. Measurements of morbidity, mortality and years of life lost are three methods used to demonstrate the inequities of health service distribution in Australian society.

Another way of describing the connection between class and illness is to say that socioeconomic status has an inverse relationship with disease and injury. The more privileged your class, the less likely you are to develop certain diseases. Health is affected most negatively by unemployment—unemployed people are the least privileged group in society. Those who are employed full-time, and women who are employed part-time, are the only groups with above average physical and mental health (ABS 1998). Many studies conclude that 'there is sufficient evidence to say that unemployment *causes* ill health . . .' (Duckett 2000, p 15). For example, the rate of illness for unemployed people is 20–30% higher than those who are employed (Germov 2002).

The burden of short- and long-term illnesses borne disproportionately by people with lower SES is not confined to physical illness and disabilities (Bruce, Takeuchi & Leaf 1991). For instance, it also appears that the mental health and social functioning of unemployed people may be significantly lower than for employed people. In one study conducted in Sydney, the women who were unemployed revealed higher levels of social exclusion (Moore et al 2003), which can result in mental health problems such as depression. Similarly, a recent study in the United Kingdom revealed an association between the prevalence of common mental disorders and low income (Weich, Lewis, & Jenkins 2001). A major Australian study of mental illness rates (Australian Bureau of Statistics (ABS) 1998) also demonstrated that unemployed people:

- are most likely to have either, or both, a physical and mental disorder;
- have the highest rate of substance abuse;
- have the highest rate of anxiety disorders; and
- have the highest rate of depression.

However, as Chris' story demonstrates, employment is no guarantee of health, for certain jobs have far higher morbidity rates than others. Chris' health problems were compounded by work-related emotional stress, but physical injury is also significant. For example, in 1992–1993, there were 24.9 injuries per 1000 workers (George & Davis 1998). Eight per cent of the workforce sustains work-based injuries each year, but they are most prevalent among general labourers (40%), metal workers (20%), miners (17%), and waterside workers (12.5%) (Burdess 1999). These are working class jobs in which men predominate. However, the wives of men who work in dusty jobs or with toxic chemicals have above average levels of cervical cancer. Air borne pollution causing or worsening disease is also experienced more by working class families who live closer to polluting factories, arterial roads, and cargo ports with high density diesel-powered truck traffic. They are also more likely to live down-wind from smoke stacks or open mines (Burdess 1999).

From the discussion so far, it is clear that people who are more affluent experience better health than poorer people (Sainsbury & Harris 2001). They also experience lower comparative mortality rates. For example, by dividing the population into five equal groups (with 20% of the population in each quintile), the class gradient for mortality is clear in all developed countries (Sainsbury & Harris 2001). All of the lower death rates apply to the 20% of the population with the highest SES, and all the higher rates relate to the poorest 20%—whose deaths from respiratory disease, stroke and heart disease are twice the expected rate (Giddens 2001). In Australia, circulatory system disease like Chris's shows the clearest impact of class on death. With the same quintiles, death rates from heart disease, from poorest to richest are: 70,000, 68,000, 58,000, 48,000, and 35,000 (Metherell 2000). That is, the poorest Australians have twice the death rate as the richest group (70,000 versus 35,000).

Years of life lost (YLL) calculations take into account the age at which a person dies. They acknowledge that early deaths (those occurring before the expected life span at a given point in time) have a greater impact upon the individual and their family. This measure is calculated from the average remaining life expectancy less 3% (Vos et al 2001). The death of a woman from breast cancer at the age of 45 would gain a higher YLL measure than a woman who dies of stroke at the age of 75, when the life expectancy of women at present is over 80 years. Similarly, the death of Chris's father at the age of 35 would result in a higher YLL measure, because of the devastating financial impact it had on his young wife and family. Vos and colleagues' (2001) Victorian research in the 1990s showed big differences in the YLL between people in each of the SES quintiles for the following causes of death: ischaemic heart disease, chronic obstructive airways disease, diabetes, asthma, sudden infant death syndrome, road traffic accidents and homicides. Every group living in a poorer area than the 20% above them show a step-by-step increase in the YLL burden per 1000 people.

What all of these morbidity and mortality calculations make clear is that the poorer a person is, the more likely it is that they will die from respiratory disease, cerebrovascular accidents, heart disease, injuries, cancer and infant deaths (Giddens 2001). In Australia, the death rates are consistently higher for those of lower SES than those with higher SES across the lifespan (Harding et al 2002).

# Access

In the past thirty years, increased health spending on accident prevention activities such as compulsory seat belts and random alcohol breath testing; and health promotion campaigns to reduce cigarette and high fat food intake, have modestly improved the health status of Australians. Ultimately however, the main health issue to be addressed at the prevention level is that of poverty, because of its flow-on effects on housing, education, nutrition, occupation and chance of employment (George & Davis 1998). Strategies to improve the circumstances of those on low incomes (and ultimately their health) are complex, in that there are higher than proportional numbers of

Indigenous people, recent immigrants and unskilled workers in the ranks of the unemployed. These groups are, as this chapter and Chapter 6 demonstrates, less healthy than the national norm, and have particular needs.

One issue is that people from lower SES backgrounds are less likely to be aware of, or understand, illness prevention measures. Similarly, they are less likely to have access to health treatments or know how to utilise them when they are available. Moore and colleagues' (2003) study of young women living in a lower class Sydney suburb showed that 40% did not use local health services because they did not know about them or they were hard to access. Poorer Australian women have significantly lower participation rates of pap smear testing for cervical cancer and mammography screening for breast cancer. Likewise, children from low-income families are less likely to be fully immunised against diphtheria, whooping cough and measles. This may not be a risk for them in the short term, but if population levels of effective immunisation fall below a certain threshold, then the whole group is at risk for these contagious diseases. The poor also use less preventative and maintenance dental care—especially since the free Commonwealth Dental Health Program was abandoned in 1997—and this ultimately leads to more tooth extractions and adverse health later in life (Burdess 1999).

Australians most affected by medical costs are those like Chris, whose income is just high enough for them to be ineligible for a health care concession card. If individuals in this group become ill, they have to locate a bulk billing general practitioner, as they cannot afford private health insurance. Those with health insurance are wealthier, better educated and older than those without (Duckett 2000). Inequities in access to health care are obvious when you realise that in 2002, the average Medicare expenditure in Australia that was rebated by the government was $530 per person per annum. Compare this to the rebate of $900 per person per annum in Double Bay, which is a wealthy Sydney suburb; and some remote Aboriginal settlements, where it was as low as $80 per annum (Metherell 2002). This pattern of higher levels of public and private health spending on richer people occurs in western countries even though they are less sick and have less chronic illnesses.

Because of the poorer health of lower income people, acute hospital admissions in 2000 in inner and western Sydney—generally lower SES suburbs—were 20% higher than average, and in more affluent suburbs 15% lower (Metherell 2002; Turrell & Mathers 2000). This indicates that the lack of awareness of, access to, and use of screening and early intervention health services means that poorer people are less protected from preventable diseases. They have illness diagnosed later; therefore, if they are hospitalised, they are sicker, harder to treat and, if the condition is not fatal, are more likely to require complex rehabilitation.

# Structured inequalities and coronary heart disease

Coronary heart disease remains the biggest single cause of death in Australia (Leeder 1999). Furthermore, in Australia, less affluent men are 54% more likely, and less affluent women are 124% more likely to die from CHD than their more privileged counterparts (Higginbotham, Albrecht & Freeman 2001). Let's have a look at how all of these issues—upstream, midstream and downstream factors; morbidity and mortality rates—can be synthesised so that we understand the contributing factors and develop some strategies for our client Chris.

First, we need to know that the increased risk for premature death from CHD is due to risk factors like cigarette smoking, obesity, and heavy alcohol consumption (Hayen et al 2002). Unfortunately, current rates of tobacco smoking continue to increase with SES disadvantage. Women and men who are unemployed, work part-time, or are unable to work, smoke at much higher rates than the average (Moore & Jorm 2001). In fact, lowest status Australians smoke cigarettes at twice the rate of those from the highest class.

Similarly, working class diets generally comprise a higher percentage of unhealthy foods like fried meat, meat products, sugar and over-refined cereals. This nutritionally poor diet is linked to obesity, hypertension and CHD. As well as eating more saturated fats, working class diets tend not to include more beneficial foods such as fresh fruit, vegetables, whole grain and low fat dairy products. It is this combination of saturated fats and refined carbohydrates with insufficient fibre and protective vitamins that leads to being overweight. In turn, being overweight and poorly nourished are major risk factors for the range of conditions Chris developed, including hypertension, atherosclerosis, and coronary heart disease.

Lower paid and middle management jobs are often more stressful because of boredom, long hours, and the realistic fear of retrenchment. People with little control over their life at work may assume they have little control over their life outside work and have low health expectations (Burdess 1999). Continuing high risk practices may also be due to lack of awareness or knowledge, insufficient money to pay for healthy food, perceived irrelevance, lack of time to exercise or access programs due to longer or more antisocial working hours, or youthful or macho beliefs in personal inviolability.

# Nursing strategies for working with people who are disadvantaged

Hayen and colleagues (2002) reviewed NSW mortality data to determine preventable deaths before the age of 75. Primary avoidable mortality consists of conditions that could be prevented through changes in individual health-related behaviours, or through population level interventions; for example, legislation to reduce general exposure to hazards such as cigarette smoke. Ischaemic heart disease was the biggest contributor to primary avoidable mortality throughout the 20 years under study. For every 100 potentially avoidable deaths from heart disease, the researchers found that half would respond to primary prevention strategies that nurses could endorse, such as stopping smoking, improving diet and increasing physical activity. Another quarter of CHD deaths could be prevented by secondary prevention strategies like lowering blood pressure and cholesterol in those with raised levels, or early signs of heart disease. Thus, routine screening would be beneficial. The remaining 25 deaths could have been avoided by prompt accurate medical diagnosis and appropriate treatment and rehabilitation (Hayen et al 2002).

Thus, Chris's heart attack could have been amongst the half of those Hayen and colleagues consider preventable. If he had stopped smoking cigarettes, decreased his consumption of fatty and sweet foods and increased his physical activity level, his risk of a heart attack would have been lower. Cholesterol screening could also have contributed to prevention by raising his awareness of his high level of CHD vulnerability and perhaps precipitating positive lifestyle changes some years before. However, it is important that we do not allow ourselves to be lulled into thinking that Chris is responsible for his ill-health because he hasn't been doing these things. Nurses would do well to consider the particular challenges facing people who experience socioeconomic disadvantage, especially in relation to adopting and maintaining healthy behaviours. The evidence presented in this chapter has clearly demonstrated that individualising responsibility for poor health is misguided. The evidence linking poorer health to socioeconomic disadvantage is clear, and leads inevitably to the need for community and societal strategies.

People who live with socioeconomic disadvantage need compassionate care from nurses. If they are treated disrespectfully, this may become yet another barrier discouraging them from accessing health care. An appreciation of the challenges confronting those who are poor is a good start and will allow nurses to be empathic and respond appropriately to the needs of those whose access to societal resources is reduced.

# Conclusion

Effective strategies to improve the health and wellbeing of disadvantaged groups, and to offset the impact of chronic illnesses, require a commitment to social justice and cross sector collaboration. While nursing plays an important part in this, nurses cannot do it alone. Hence, education systems, welfare and housing providers, employers, and public transport bodies all have roles to play to increase structural support for Australians in poverty. As childhood illness is highest amongst those in lower socioeconomic groups and poor childhood health predicts greater mortality and morbidity in adulthood, the wellbeing of children and mothers is fundamental to the health of our society. Good, culturally appropriate health care depends on policies that offer equal health opportunities for all regardless of income and increased funding for more upstream (preventative and population level) health and community services.

# Tutorial questions

1. What class do you belong to? How do you believe your class, ethnicity, and your gender has influenced your understanding of:
   a) health;
   b) healthy food;
   c) the importance of exercise; and
   d) substance use?

2. In countries like Australia, why do you think that many people from the working class, and some wealthy people, call themselves middle class?

3. During the last 25 years, Australian life expectancy from birth (in 1997) for men has increased by 8 years to 76, and by 6.5 years to 81.5 for women. Given this, why should nurses be concerned about health inequalities in Australia?

4. List as many downstream, middle stream and upstream factors you can that contribute to deaths from:
   (a) cardiovascular disease;
   (b) lung cancer; and
   (c) work-related incidents.

# References

Australian Bureau of Statistics (ABS) 1998 *Mental Health and Wellbeing Profile of Adults Australia*. ABS, Canberra

Bruce ML, Takeuchi DT, Leaf P J 1991 Poverty and psychiatric status. *Archives of General Psychiatry* 48:470–474

Burdess N 1999 Class and health. In: Grbich C (ed), *Health in Australia*, 2nd edn. Longman, Sydney, pp 149–171

Drevdahl D, Kneipp SM, Canales MK, Dorcy KS 2001 Reinvesting in social justice: A capital idea for public health nursing. *Advances in Nursing Science* 24(2):19–31

Duckett SJ 2000 *The Australian Health Care System*. Oxford University Press, Melbourne

Germov J 2002 Class, health inequality, and social justice. In: Germov J (ed), *Second Opinion. An Introduction to Health Sociology*, 2nd edn. Oxford University Press, pp 67–94

George J, Davies A 1998 *States of Health. Health and Illness in Australia*, 3rd edn. Longman, Sydney

Giddens A 2001 *Sociology*, 4th edn. Polity Press, Cambridge

Gorman C 2003 The no.1 killer of women. *Time*. April 28, pp 51–6

Harding A, Lloyd R, Greenwell H 2002 *Financial Disadvantage in Australia 1990 to 2000. The persistence of Poverty in a Decade of Growth*, National Centre for Social and Economic Modelling, Canberra

Hayen A, Lincoln D, Moore H, Thomas M 2002 Trends in potentially avoidable mortality in NSW, *NSW Public Health Journal* 13:226–241

Higginbotham N, Albrecht G, Freeman S 2001 Heart disease in transdisciplinary perspective. In: N Higginbotham, G Albrecht & L Connor (eds), *Health Social*

*Science. A Transdisciplinary and Complex Perspective.* Oxford University Press, Melbourne, pp 93–114

Horton R 2003 Commentary. Medical journals: evidence of bias against diseases of poverty. *The Lancet* 361:712–713

Kivimaki M, Leino-Arjas P, Luukkoven R, Riihimaki H, Vahtera J, Kirjonen J 2002 Work stress and risk of cardiovascular mortality: prospective cohort study of industrial employees. *British Medical Journal* 325:857–860

Leeder S 1999 *Healthy Medicine, Challenges Facing Australia's Health Services.* Allen & Unwin, Sydney

Marmot M 2000 Social determinants of health: from observation to policy. *Medical Journal of Australia* 172:379–380

Metherell M 2000 Health link to income on the rise. The *Sydney Morning Herald*, May 15, p 7

Metherell M 2002 Call to lift staff to beat health crisis. The *Sydney Morning Herald.* June 25, p 4

Moore H, Jorm L 2001 Measuring health inequalities in New South Wales. *NSW Public Health Journal* 12:120–125.

Moore M, Lane D, Kroon V, Griffiths R, Horsfall J 2003 *Villawood Icebreakers: a Program for Community Development. Survey Report I.* South Western Sydney Area Health Service & the University of Western Sydney, Sydney

Sainsbury P, Harris E 2001 Health inequalities: something old, something new. *NSW Public Health Journal* 12:117–119

Turrell G 2002 Reducing socioeconomic health inequalities: issues of relevance for policy. *NSW Public Health Journal* 13:47–49

Turrell G, Mathers CD 2000 Socioeconomic status and health in Australia. *Medical Journal of Australia* 172:434–438

Vos T, Begg S, Chen Y, Magnus A 2001 Socioeconomic differentials in life expectancy and years of life lost in Victoria, 1992–1996. *NSW Public Health Journal* 12:126–130

Weich S, Lewis G, Jenkins SP, 2001 Income inequality and the prevalence of common mental disorders in Britain. *British Journal of Psychiatry* 178:222–227

# Chapter 4

## Gender and Health

*Cath Rogers-Clark, Wendy Lee Kyle and Geoff Wilson*

**This chapter:**

- introduces the concept of 'gender' as a powerful factor influencing the health status of women and men;
- explores how being female can influence a woman's pattern of health and illness;
- outlines and discusses significant women's health problems;
- overviews the evidence about men's health status in Australia; and
- considers the influence of biological, cultural and social factors on men's health.

This chapter considers how being female or male influences a person's health status. There is clear evidence that gender is an important factor in determining the amount of illness, the sorts of diseases and the life expectancy of an individual. Gender is not the only, nor necessarily the most important factor in determining health status, but its influence is pervasive. This chapter gives insights into the health experiences of both men and women, and provides analyses of the ways in which gender can influence these health experiences.

The stories of Sara and Warren are used to provide 'real life' examples of the main points made in this chapter. Their stories are not necessarily 'typical' of all women and men but they do highlight some of the common health issues affecting each gender.

## The health of women

What does being female mean in terms of a woman's health across her lifetime? Will it affect the sorts of diseases she could suffer? Secondly, could her gender mean that a woman experiences wellness and illness differently from men, and receives different health care than a man? This section will endeavour to answer these two questions. To illustrate the main points of the chapter, we will refer to Sara's health experiences. Sara is a 51-year-old woman, living in regional Australia.

## Case study

Sara has had her share of good and bad times. She's been divorced for the past five years, having escaped her violent marriage, which had lasted for twenty years. Her children, Tania and Jodie, are teenagers and attending the local high school. Sara works thirty hours a week as a nurse in the local aged care facility. She'd like to do some study to upgrade her qualifications but it's expensive so she hasn't been able to.

Sara's health has been reasonable. She suffered a few problems, which her GP says are due to her beginning menopause, but they are manageable. She does find that it's hard to manage her weight, though, and whilst her GP has asked her to follow a low-fat diet, start exercising and quit smoking, Sara has always found that easier said than done. She is really busy managing work as well as being a sole parent, and can never find time to get out and exercise. She tries to prepare healthy food at home, but the kids won't eat it and so she finds it easier to cook the foods she knows they will eat. As for giving up smoking, well that seems just too difficult. She's been smoking since she was 15 and says she'll probably die with a cigarette in her hand because she's so addicted. In the last year or two she's been avoiding going to her GP, because she knows she'll get nagged again about all that.

Recently, Sara has been experiencing some chest pain during the night. She decided it was probably indigestion and so didn't do anything about it but her children pressured her into going to her GP, who said it was probably stress-related. A couple of weeks later she experienced such severe pain that she panicked and got her kids to call an ambulance. It turns out she was having a heart attack. Not a big one, according to the doctors at the hospital, but enough of one to be a real warning.

## How being female affects the health and illness patterns of women

Many readers would realise that, on average, women live longer than men in many parts of the world. This is certainly the case in all developed countries, although there are a few noteworthy exceptions. In a few countries in South Asia, such as Bangladesh and Nepal, men have longer life spans than women (Cockerham 2004).

Why do women in most parts of the world live longer than men, and has this always been the case? The evidence available to us suggests that in pre-industrial times, women and men lived to approximately the same age. This situation continued until relatively recently; in the 1850s, in England and Wales for example, both men and women had a life expectancy of around

59 years (Cockerham 2004). However in the early 1900s this picture changed, and the gap between the average woman's and the average man's lifespan increased to the point where, for example, as a group, Australian women live more than five years longer than Australian men. There is some evidence now that this gap may have peaked and could be shrinking (Cockerham 2004). Possible causes for this include women's increasing uptake of traditionally male pursuits, including wider commitment to having a successful career (and the stresses that come with it, especially when combined with the traditional women's work of caring for family), and cigarette smoking.

An interesting paradox within women's health is that, whilst women do live longer than men, they also consistently report more illness and a poorer health-related quality of life than men. In other words, they appear to get sick more often, and the symptoms associated with their sickness can reduce their life enjoyment. For example, in the 2001 Health Survey, 21% of women reported suffering arthritis, as compared to 15% of men (ABS 2003), whilst 12.2% of women said they had experienced a mental or behavioural problem, as compared to 8.7% of men.

There are a variety of factors contributing to this apparent paradox. One is that women may be more willing to acknowledge their illnesses and seek help than men. For example, in 2001 it was estimated that 27% of females had consulted a doctor in the previous two weeks, compared with 21% of males (ABS 2003).

The second factor is that the diseases which more often afflict women cause suffering but not necessarily death. The opposite is true for men. They report fewer non life-threatening conditions, but are more likely to be grappling with life-threatening conditions. For example, in the 2001 Health Survey, 2.5% of the men who participated said they currently had cancer, compared to 1.8% of women (ABS 2003).

The third factor is the nature of women's lives, as opposed to men's. Whilst there have been significant changes in women's lives in the past forty years, driven particularly by the second wave of feminism begun in the 1960s, there continue to be significant differences between how men and women live. For example, women continue to do the bulk of unpaid caring for children, the elderly and the disabled, and there is evidence that women find the 'superwoman' expectations overwhelming (Pretty 1998). These expectations lead women to believe that they must be successful in domesticity, the traditional female domain, whilst also excelling in the male dominated domain of work (Novack & Novack 1996, Philpot et al 1997). These dual sets of expectations create high levels of stress for women who are working and managing a home and family, or caring for elderly or disabled relatives, as well as a lack of time to engage in self-care activities such as exercise and relaxation. Sara's recent heart attack fits with this picture. As a sole parent she's found it difficult to find time to manage work and home life. This has left her very little time to take care of herself by preparing healthy food and taking regular exercise which, coupled with her long-term smoking habit, has no doubt increased her vulnerability to cardiovascular disease.

Although the evidence suggests that women do experience more ill health than men, there appears to be no significant difference between men's and women's perceptions of their health status. In 2001, the majority of Australians aged 15 years and over perceived themselves as being in good health, with 82% reporting their health as good, very good or excellent (ABS 2003). This suggests that overall, whilst women appear to experience more health concerns, these concerns do not jeopardise women's perceptions of their own health and wellbeing.

# Common women's health issues

Often, discussion of 'women's health' leads to a discussion about women's reproductive health. After all, women's reproductive functions lead to bodily experiences such as menarche, menstruation, fertility, pregnancy, childbirth, breastfeeding and menopause. Health problems related to women's reproductive functions are diverse and include such things as dysmenorrhoea (painful periods), sexually transmissible illnesses leading to chronic problems such as pelvic inflammatory disease and infertility, birth-related problems, mastitis (a common infection of the breast tissue in women who are breastfeeding) and cancers of the breast, uterus, cervix and ovaries.

The list of reproductive-related women's health problems is quite long, and perhaps it's not surprising that 'women's health' is often thought to be synonymous with women's reproductive health. At times, this analogy is relevant. Later in this chapter there is a discussion about obstetric fistulae, a serious women's reproductive health issue affecting many women from underdeveloped countries, who lack access to the type of maternity care to which women from western societies have ready access. As you will read later, women who live with obstetric fistulae have a profoundly reduced quality of life because of this problem.

Despite the range of women's health concerns related to their reproductive functioning, women also face a myriad of health problems which are not related. Health problems unrelated to reproductive health are more likely to be the cause of morbidity and mortality in women. For example, an editorial in the influential medical journal *Lancet* recently identified heart attacks and stroke as the 'greatest threat to women's health' on a worldwide basis (2003, p 1165). Twice as many women die from cardiovascular disease as from all forms of cancer, and women are more likely to die from cardiovascular disease than men.

This may be surprising for some readers, because it is contrary to 'common knowledge'. Heart disease is generally viewed as a problem affecting men, and tends to conjure images of middle-aged men having sudden and sometimes fatal heart attacks. Even amongst health professionals, there has been a perception that women do not get heart disease prior to menopause, despite evidence to the contrary (Miracle 2004). As you will recall from Sara's story, she was unconcerned when she first experienced chest pain, thinking that it was just indigestion. Obviously the thought that she might have heart disease had not occurred to her, even though she is a nurse.

Of particular concern is that this lack of awareness is also evident amongst health professionals. Research suggests that women may receive less thorough and less intensive investigations of their cardiovascular symptoms than men (Ayanian & Epstein 1991, Miracle 2004, Steingart et al 1991). In the first instance, this happened to Sara, whose GP did not consider the possibility that Sara might have heart disease at such a relatively young age. This failure to assess women's cardiovascular symptoms with the same vigour as when they occur in men could stem from the pervasive belief that heart disease is not as dangerous for women as it if for men (Broom 2002). In this scenario, we see the dangers of assuming that reproductive health is the key component of women's health.

## Women's roles, women's lives, women's health

There are significant differences around the world in relation to the health of women. In Australia and other developing countries, the health of women has markedly improved over time and this is related to better nutrition, access to clean water, sewage systems, better health care, and so on. In the past twenty-five years, since the beginning of the women's health movement, the health needs of women have received special attention, with a suite of women's health services targeting particular health problems as well as selected groups of women. For example, in Sara's home town in regional Australia, specialist women's health services include a young women's service targeting young disadvantaged women and girls with a specialist antenatal and postnatal service; three breast cancer diagnostic clinics; and a women's health nurse service.

This is not necessarily the case worldwide. The health of women, men and children everywhere around the world is linked to their financial status, but the social roles and status of men and women also play a major role. The health of women is linked strongly to the status of women, and this is very evident in countries where women occupy a lesser position in society than men. As the World Health Organization states in its *Gender Policy* (2002, p 1):

> Society prescribes to women and men different roles in different social contexts. There are also differences in the opportunities and resources available to women and men, and in their ability to make decisions and exercise their human rights, including those related to protecting health and seeking care in case of ill health. Gender roles and unequal gender relations interact with other social and economic variables, resulting in different and sometimes inequitable patterns of exposure to health risk, and in differential access to and utilization of health information, care and services.

The example of obstetric fistula in women in developing countries provides compelling evidence of this link. Obstetric fistula is a health problem caused by obstructed labour in birthing women. When the baby's head is pushed against the woman's pelvis for a long period of time, death of the surrounding tissue can result. This can cause a hole to form between the woman's bladder and vagina, leading to urinary incontinence, or between the rectum and vagina, leading to faecal incontinence. Usually, the woman's baby is stillborn. For women, the consequences of obstetric fistulae are tragic.

They have lost their baby, they smell bad because of their incontinence, and are often shunned by their husbands, families and communities (Donnay & Weil 2004).

In developed countries, high quality midwifery and obstetric care means that obstetric fistulae rarely occur. Yet, over two million women worldwide have this problem (Murray & Lopez 1998). It is caused by malnutrition, generally poor health, and early marriage leading to pregnancy before physiological maturity (Donnay & Weil 2004). Early marriage is related to lack of education. Girls who have the opportunity to go to school delay having children, and this reduces their risk of developing obstetric fistulae (Bangser, Gumodoka & Berege 1999). Furthermore, many women living with obstetric fistulae usually are not aware that surgical treatment is effective in resolving the problem and, even if they are aware, are unlikely to have access to this treatment.

# Violence against women

Another significant women's health issue highlighted by governments, community groups and women themselves is violence against women. Violence against women can involve the threat or use of physical violence to frighten or harm a woman; or sexual assault, which is any sexual act forced upon a woman without her consent (ABS 2002). Violence against women is strongly linked to perceptions of a woman's 'place' in society. The United Nations Declaration on the 'Elimination of Violence Against Women' noted that it is a symptom of unequal power relationships between men and women, and is a primary violation of basic human rights (Oswomen 1992).

A survey in 1996 revealed that 7% of Australian women (490,400) had experienced at least one incidence of violence in the past twelve months, with 404,400 of these women reporting physical violence and 133,100 reporting sexual violence. Women were over four times more likely to be assaulted by a man than by a woman. A particularly distressing finding was that 22% of women (109,100) reported that more than one perpetrator had abused them in the preceding twelve months (ABS 2002).

Nurses and other health professionals need to be aware that a woman's response to recent or past violence can lead to mental and physical health problems such as insomnia, anxiety, eating disorders, depression and suicide attempts, headaches or heart palpitations (Anderson, Harris & Madl 1998). Violence against men by men is also common, and of concern. However, violence against women by men is particularly traumatic because it is characterised by an abuse of power, which usually occurs within the confines of a relationship or at the time of separation due to relationship failure. Sara says that her abuse started when she was pregnant with Tania. Her husband could be a kind and generous partner, but when he drank too much alcohol his whole personality changed and this led to him hitting her. In the beginning this happened rarely, but as the years went by it happened a lot more often. Sara loved her husband, and was scared because she didn't know how she would cope on her own, but eventually she could see that her children were being badly affected. With the help of the local domestic violence service, Sara was able to gather her strength to leave her husband and begin life again. This took a couple of years because she was suffering from depression and needed a lot of support to believe in herself again.

Violence against women is difficult to identify and respond to because it is hidden. Research indicates that women who have been abused do seek the assistance of health professionals in treating their injuries, but are unlikely to reveal the cause of these injuries for a variety of reasons (Anderson, Harris & Madl 1998). Health professionals often do not detect that violence has occurred and, even if they are aware, do not always respond appropriately. Sara recalls that once, when she sought help at the local hospital after a particularly bad bashing, one of her nurses gave her a lecture about how she should just leave her marriage. One of the most common myths surrounding domestic violence is that women should find it easy to simply leave the violent relationship. The reality is that women find it very difficult to do so. This may be because they are afraid that their partner will pursue them and injure them further; because they love their partners and want the violence to stop but not their relationship; because they lack financial resources; or because they stay to keep an intact family for their children. If health professionals act in disparaging ways to women who choose to stay with their violent partners, those women are unlikely to return for follow-up care.

## Women's roles, women's lives, women's health care

We have noted the mistaken assumption that women's health is largely synonymous with women's reproductive functioning, which derives from the notion that a woman's biology determines her destiny. Along with their distinguishing biology, women are also considered to have a variety of other characteristics, such as being emotional, dependent, caring, illogical and intuitive (George & Davis 1998). Whether these characteristics do emanate from women's biology or whether they actually arise from differential socialisation and role expectations continues to be debated but, regardless of this, these assumed characteristics underpin the role and status of women. In our society, despite women's increasing participation in higher education, professional and business men largely continue their hold over the reins of political and corporate power. Women in turn continue to perform most of the unpaid caring work within families, often whilst simultaneously undertaking paid work. Sara has this experience. As a sole parent she is working hard in her paid work as well as being singularly responsible for raising her children.

Beliefs about women permeate the health professions and influence the health care offered to women. A belief that women are more emotional and illogical than men, for example, can lead to the inappropriate diagnosis of emotional health problems in women and subsequent over-prescription of medications such as tranquillisers. Mental health workers may consider that emotional distress and problem behaviours in a woman are signs of 'madness', whereas these behaviours in men are more likely to be viewed as indicative of 'badness' (Creedy & Nizette 1998). A tendency to assume that emotional health problems are common in women can be dangerous for women. In Sara's case, her GP incorrectly thought that Sara's chest pain was stress-related and as we've already seen this was not the case.

One of the major contributions of the women's health movement over the past thirty years has been to sensitise health professionals to women's needs when accessing health care. There has been considerable evidence collected that demonstrates that medical practitioners in particular were offering women sub-standard care. Sexism in medicine has been demonstrated by the failure to conduct research on women's health issues; not informing women of the treatment options available to them, or of the side-effects of their treatments; and inappropriately labelling their health concerns as psychosomatic (Broome 2002). The advent of specialist women's health centres provided a showcase for a model of women's health care that provided accessible and appropriate health services for women. Women's health centres emphasised a partnership model of care, where women were fully informed and made their own choices with information and support from the professional staff (Rogers-Clark 1998). In the early years of women's health centres (the 1970s onwards) this model of care was in stark contrast to that offered by mainstream health services. Since then it is evident that mainstream health services for women have adopted many of the principles of women-centred care, in response to the very clear messages from many groups of women calling for such reforms. Despite her GP's incorrect diagnosis, Sara thinks highly of her. She says that her GP is friendly, down to earth and listens to her side of the story. She always asks Sara what she would like to do about any health concern she has, rather than simply telling her what she should do.

## Summary

This section has demonstrated that being female is likely to have a significant impact on a woman's experience of health and illness. In general, women live longer than men, but length of life is not necessarily accompanied by quality of life, because women in general experience more ill health than men. Reproductive health issues are of course important for women, but cardiovascular disease is the biggest cause of premature death of women worldwide. The place of women in society is fundamentally tied to their health experiences. Health services have been guilty of failing to respond appropriately to women's health needs in countries where women's status is low; and in western societies women have complained that their health concerns have been marginalised, poorly diagnosed or inappropriately treated. These complaints have led to a new focus on the formulation of health partnerships with women, emphasising equity between patient and provider, choice, and informed decision-making.

Are the same factors important in men's health? The next section explores just that question.

# The health of men

This section will review the effects of gender on men's health and illness experiences. It is important for health professionals to understand why men appear, in general, to have worse health outcomes than women (McMurray 1999, p 217). The women's health movement helped to highlight the contribution of gender as a key factor underpinning experiences of health and illness. In response, it is now evident that a gender analysis of men's health experiences, previously overlooked by practitioners, academics and policy makers, is equally important. Evidence of this need can be drawn from a simple examination of life expectancy rates, where currently in Australia the life expectancy for men is 77 years as compared to 82.4 for women (ABS 2001).

As with women's health, a limitation of the mainstream health services offered to men has been their predominant biomedical focus. Medical conditions associated with heart disease, respiratory disease, diabetes mellitus and cerebrovascular disease, as well as gender specific conditions such as prostate disease, impotency and testicular cancer have received the most attention. This is despite compelling evidence that, in Australia, and overseas, the rates of stress, accidental death through motor vehicle accident, drowning, risk taking activities and suicide (particularly in the age groups 15–24 and 75–79) are higher for men than women. Poor food habits, obesity, alcohol consumption and smoking are also more common in men than women and are major contributors to their shortened life expectancy (ABS 2001; White & Cash 2003).

Within Australia, and overseas, the past ten years has seen a groundswell of men's health research, health programs and policy development. In general, these initiatives have emphasised a holistic approach to men's health which acknowledges that many of the most serious men's health issues are strongly affected by gender issues.

## Case study

Warren, a 42-year-old man, had recently participated in an unplanned shopping centre health assessment, which revealed a variety of negative health indicators. He shared these results with his general practitioner, but only after strong encouragement from his wife. He was obese with a body mass index of 35, smoked approximately 25 cigarettes daily, and was sedentary in his habits. His resting blood pressure was found to be in the hypertensive range of 145/95 mmHg, and his serum cholesterol was significantly elevated.

He reported that his marriage had been under strain due to his long working hours as an accountant, and he had little time to spend with his two teenage children. He said that he and his wife were now separated but that he hoped that they would be able to resume their relationship once they'd had some time to 'cool off'.

Warren's GP convinced him to enter a Cardiovascular Rehabilitation Program. Warren's personal goals on entering the program were to lose weight, stop smoking, increase his cardiovascular fitness, and lower his cholesterol, as well as learn to handle stress more effectively. Half way through the program, he had reduced his cholesterol and weight slightly, but had not been able to change his stress levels and was still smoking. The cardiac rehabilitation nurse noted in Warren's chart that he seemed unresponsive in his stress management sessions. He constantly joked through the sessions, and did not engage in the 'homework' activities set for him in relation to learning relaxation techniques.

Warren is a middle-aged Aussie 'bloke', and his story is, in our experience, not uncommon. Men like Warren may have been socialised and conditioned to believe that they should be in control and able to take care of themselves, reinforcing, to a large degree, that they are invincible and should not rely on others for help. This is the 'She'll be right mate' approach (Department of Veteran's Affairs 2000), which is often seen as representative of Australian men. Whether this particular approach to life is in fact representative of most Australian men will be debated later in this chapter. The major message to take from this case study is that Warren's health has a lot to do with his work role, his relationship, and how he thinks about his health.

## Theorising gender differences in health

Why is it that men and women experience different levels of health and illness? Generally, gender health differences are assumed to be due to biological factors, behavioural and cultural factors, or material/structural factors (Woods 2001).

Biological factors could influence men's health in a variety of ways. The first is that male babies are more fragile than female babies. More male embryos are conceived than female embryos; however the male foetus is more vulnerable to death and damage than female babies. Perinatal brain damage, cerebral palsy, some congenital deformities, and premature birth and stillbirth are more common in boys (Kraemer 2000). Another theory linking biology to men's health behaviour is that testosterone, which increases aggressiveness and sexual drive in men, is also responsible for men's lack of responsiveness to their own needs, since their biology directs them to be focused outwards rather than inwards. It is certainly true that the withholding of emotions such as fear and anxiety was beneficial for a male in the past when on the hunt, but clearly this no longer applies in modern society. Overall, however, there is a lack of clear evidence that biology strongly influences the status of men's health, and it is thought that social factors cause the most significant variation in health status between different groups in society (Wood 2001).

In relation to behavioural and cultural explanations, there has been a great deal of speculation that the traditional male gender role is closely linked to men's attitudes and behaviours in relation to their own health. Within this so-called 'typical' gender role, men are discouraged from complaining about their circumstances and speaking out to others about their needs. Instead, hallmarks of the traditional male role include being dominant, being in control, being competitive, and being preoccupied with work (Huggins 1995). Whilst there is a common perception amongst health professionals and within the community that this traditional men's role is responsible for many of the 'problematic' behaviours which put men at risk of poorer health, in fact this view may not be true for all men. Certainly Warren appears to represent this particular form of masculinity. As we saw earlier in the chapter, Warren works hard and this appears to have led to some major relationship problems for him. We also sense that Warren felt uncomfortable with the 'stress management' component of his cardiac rehabilitation program, despite his desire to reduce his stress levels. It's possible that focusing on his feelings caused Warren some distress, which he chose to 'cover up' with attempts at humour.

Whilst we focus on Warren as meeting the requirements of the 'traditional male gender role', it is most important to acknowledge very clearly that men are not all the same! There is significant evidence from historians and anthropologists that there is not a singular form of masculinity but rather a number of 'masculinities' in existence (Connell et al 1998). Whilst some boys and men embrace a traditional view of masculinity, others express their masculinity differently. Men from different cultures, age groups, geographical locations and social classes may be quite different in their key values and attitudes, and ways of living. In Australia for example, there are large communities of Greek, Italian, Lebanese and Vietnamese peoples, to name just a few. These communities have their own gender practices developed over time (Connell et al 1998). Even within relatively homogenous groups, there will be significant differences between the men and/or boys of these groups.

It is vital to consider the implications of 'multiple masculinities' when devising men's health programs and strategies, which are likely to have limited success if they are devised using a common view of masculinity. There are significant groups of men who are disadvantaged in terms of their health, including Indigenous men, men from non-English speaking backgrounds, homosexual men, men from rural and remote communities, men who live in poverty and men with disabilities (Connell et al 1998). These groups of men require targeted interventions built on a firm understanding of their particular health concerns and needs.

Behavioural and cultural factors may contribute to our understanding of the differences in mortality/morbidity in relation to 'risk taking'. Men are more likely to experience an accidental injury or death than women (Cockerham 2004), related in part to their higher involvement in risk-taking behaviours such as excessive alcohol consumption and illicit drug abuse (Davies et al 2000). Men also face occupational risks, given their high representation in workplaces that are known to have higher rates of workplace injuries, such as building sites, mining, or indeed the battlefield. (Connell et al 1998).

The degree to which a man is integrated within his community is also linked to a number of men's health issues. Socially isolated people get sick and die more readily than people who have good networks of support (Quick & Wilkinson 1991). The implication here is that people who feel they belong to a society or community, and also feel they have emotional and physical support from that community, have better health and longevity. For example, Wilson (1995) found that men reported better levels of compliance with healthy lifestyle when their primary support networks were intact. This is problematic for Warren, who is newly separated from his wife. For a start, there were the day-to-day difficulties of taking care of himself. His wife had always done most of the cooking and cleaning at home because he was so busy at work. Warren found that he was relying on takeaway food too much, and told the nurse at the cardiac rehabilitation clinic that he knew he was 'getting into the grog', particularly at night, because evenings on his own seemed almost unbearable.

There is some evidence that men are particularly traumatised, and have difficulty coping, when their primary relationship ends. For example, men's suicide rate during the time of a relationship breakdown is fifteen times that of women during the same period. A possible reason for this astonishing figure is that in over 90% of cases, children remain with their mothers when a relationship ends (Hart 1996). Coupled with the loss of the home, and often restricted access to children, a man may feel an overwhelming sense of grief. The cardiac rehabilitation nurse sensed that Warren was not doing so well, and asked him to stay back and have a chat after a session. Despite his earlier reluctance to talk about his feelings, Warren felt so relieved that someone was prepared to listen to him. He had some mates at work, but they never really talked about private matters. Sometimes he felt as if it was all too much and he didn't know how to keep going. That thought scared him.

Employment may be another key factor in determining men's health and wellbeing. Loss of, or inability to gain, employment may lessen a males' self-esteem and set the scene for depression, with its concomitant spiralling mental, emotional, physical and spiritual impact on their health status (Hart 1996). Fortunately, Warren was able to rely on his work to help him through his tough times. At least he could feel good about himself there. He liked achieving things, and got a great sense of satisfaction from a job well done. Unemployed men do not have this outlet.

Material and social factors constitute the third category of likely causes for the differences in women's and men's health status (Woods 2001). Overall, Australian men and women are, on international standards, very healthy with indicators such as life expectancy showing that our health is continuing to improve (Australian Institute of Health and Welfare 2002). However this 'overall' approach masks the fact that social factors such as class, employment status and ethnicity are correlated with differential health outcomes within different groups of men and women. High-risk groups include men from a low socioeconomic status and men from racial minorities (Connell et al 1998). Men with a low socioeconomic status suffer a number of conditions with more frequency in comparison to men from higher socioeconomic groups. For example, men from a lower socioeconomic background suffer ischaemic heart disease 54% more often than men from a high socioeconomic background (Woods 2002). Australian Indigenous men live, on average, 22 years less than non-Indigenous Australian men (Wenitong 2001), and experience higher levels of eye disease, respiratory disease, smoking, alcoholism and reduced access to health services (Connell et al 1998). When considering these statistics, it is important to note the compounding effect of social disadvantage, whereby the effects of a specific group membership become difficult to discern. For example, it can be difficult to unravel whether an Indigenous man's poor health is due to his race or his socioeconomic status. Chapter 3, Class, Poverty and Illness: Intersecting Links, considers the impact of socioeconomic class on health and provides a useful accompaniment to this discussion.

# Men's health beliefs and behaviours

Despite evidence that at least some groups of men are highly vulnerable to poor health, the vast majority of men report that they perceive themselves to be in good health (ABS 2003). So what do men perceive health to be? In one study of men in regional Australia, participants said that health for them was a state whereby life is enjoyed and the individual is able to fulfil their various roles. Being healthy for them related to either 'freedom from pain', 'not to be sick' or being 'free from major health problems' (Wilson 1995). The next question to consider relates to the health practices used by men to stay well.

The Australian Medical Association (AMA) believes that a good relationship with the family doctor is vital for men, acknowledging that they need a mixture of biomedical, psychological and spiritual care (1999). There is clear evidence that men visit their doctors less often than women, and this is an international phenomenon. For example, a North American study (Ted 1995) revealed that, during their middle years (44–64), men visited their doctor slightly more than half as much as women of a similar age did. In Australia, one in four Australian men did not visit a doctor within a 12-month timeframe (Glasson 2003).

Men may not make health a priority. In a study of men in rural Queensland, Jones (1996) reported results indicating that health was very rarely nominated as important in the lives of the men in his study, and that attending their general practitioner usually only occurred if their wives or other family members 'made them go'. This was the case with Warren. Some insight into why this might be so was gained through Wright's survey of Australian men (1999), with survey results revealing that men put off going to their general practitioner because they were not happy about having to wait to see the doctor, and they felt uncomfortable being at the surgery. Warren said this about going to his GP:

> I haven't been to the Doc for years . . . don't really know him to be honest. I suppose I was a bit scared at what he'd say to me too. And all that waiting. You know I just don't have time for that.

Men's role in the paid workforce may also create barriers preventing men from accessing health services. Michael Hart (1996) has suggested that the majority of men still work a full-time working week, and this has often meant that despite the onset of flexible working hours men are often expected to work longer hours without appropriate remuneration. This may mean that men do not have access to many of the health services, including health awareness and disease prevention programs, simply because they are at work when these programs are held. For example, in one regional health service, two excellent seminars on suicide were scheduled on a weekday.

# Summary

It is evident that nurses and other health professions who focus on men's health issues from a biomedical perspective fail to acknowledge that men's experiences of health and illness are embedded within their sociocultural context. Key factors to be considered in any analysis of men's health include the influence of biology, cultural and social factors on the health of men. Policy makers and clinicians need to work together to develop strategies to respond to the overall reluctance of men to access health services.

# Tutorial questions

1. Reflect on the ways in which being male or female has influenced your life to this point.

2. Consider your own health beliefs and behaviours. To what degree has your gender influenced these?

3. After reviewing the case studies in this chapter, can you recall a woman or man you have known or cared for who experienced similar situations?

   a) What were their circumstances?

   b) What things did they have in common/that differed from those faced by Sara and Warren?

   c) Identify some practical strategies and resources that could be applied to assist them to work through their challenges and achieve a positive, individualised health outcome.

# References

Anderson D, Harris, M, Madl R 1998 Women and violence. In: Rogers-Clark C. Smith A (eds) *Women's Health: A Primary Health Care Approach*. McLennan & Petty, Sydney

Australian Bureau of Statistics 2001 Health related actions-consultation with health professionals, National Health Survey, Summary of Results. Australia.Online. September 2003 <http://www.abs.gov.au/ausstats/abs@.nsf/Lookup/CACIA34167E36CA2568A90>

Australian Bureau of Statistics 2002 *Year Book Australia 2002*, ABS, Canberra. Online. 1 February 2004 <http://www.abs.gov.au/ausstats/abs@.nsf/Lookup/75F98215A758B2AACA256CE60020BA26>

Australian Bureau of Statistics 2003, *Year Book Australia 2003*, ABS, Canberra. Online. 1 February 2004 <http://www.abs.gov.au/ausstats/abs@.nsf/Lookup/4F7D3CEC8F06A9F5CA256CAD001F1393>

Australian Institute of Health and Welfare 2002, *Australia's Health 2002*, AIHW, Canberra. Online. 17 March 2004 <http://www.aihw.gov.au/publications/index.cfm?type=detail&id=7637>

Australian Medical Association 1999, Doctors denounce the 'macho myth'. Australian Medical Association Media Release. In: Healey J (ed) *Issues in Society: Mens Health*. Spinney Press, Sydney

Ayanian JZ, Epstein AM 1991 *Difference is the use of procedures between men and women*. National Men's Health Conference, AGPS, Canberra, pp 100–111

Bangser M, Gumodoka B, Berege Z 1999 A comprehensive approach to vesico-vaginal fistula: a project in Mwanza, Tanzania. In: M Berer, Ravindram T (eds) *Safe Motherhood Initiatives: Critical Issues*, Blackwell Science, Oxford

Broom D 2002 Gender and Health. In: Germov J (ed), *Second Opinion: An Introduction to Health Sociology*, 2nd edn. Oxford, Melbourne

Cockerham WC 2004 *Medical Sociology*, 9th edn. Pearson Prentice Hall, New Jersey

Connell RW, Schofield T, Walker L, Wood J, Butland DL, Fisher J, Bowyer J 1998 *Men's Health: A Research Agenda and Background Report*, AGPS, Canberra

Creedy D & Nizette D 1998, 'Women and mental illness'. In: C. Rogers-Clark & A. Smith (eds), *Women's Health: A Primary Health Care Approach*. McLennan & Petty, Sydney

Davies J, Frank J, Dochnahl A, Pickering T, Wilson K 2000 Identifying male college students' perceived health needs, barriers to seeking help, and recommendations to help men adopt healthier lifestyles. *Journal of American College Health* 48:259–268

Department of Veteran's Affairs 2000 Being a Digger and a Bloke. Online. March 18 2004 <http://www.dva.gov.au/health/menshealth/digger.htm>

Donnay, F, Weil, L 2004 Obstetric fistula: The international response. *Lancet* 363:71–72

George, J, Davis, A 1998 *States of Health: Health and Illness in Australia*, 3rd edn. Addison Wesley Longman, Sydney

Glasson, B 2003 AMA urges Aussie blokes to visit their GP in 2004. AMA Media Release. Online. April 5 2004, <http://www.ama.com.au/web.nsf/doc/WEEN-5UHVTZ>

Hart M 1996 Comments on the Draft National Men's Health Policy, Response to Draft National Men's Health Policy. Online. 6th September 2003, <http://members.ozemail.com.au/~irgeo/mhmhb.htm>

Huggins A 1995 *The Australian Male: Illness, Injury and Death by Socialisation*. Men's Health Teaching and Research Unit, Curtin University, Perth

Huggins A 1999 The Australian male: Illness, injury and death by socialisation. In: Laws T (ed), *Promoting Men's Health: An Essential Book for Nurses*, Ausmed Publications, Melbourne

Jones J 1996 Understanding health: The background to a study of men's perception of health. Proceedings of the Third Australian Rural and Remote Health Scientific Conference, Toowoomba, Australia

Kraemer S 2000 The fragile male. *British Medical Journal* 321(7276):1609–1613

Lancet Editorial 2003 The greatest threat to women's health. *Lancet* 362(9361):1165

Margo J 2003 Cancer Test: an expert refusal. *The Australian Financial Review*, 6 February, p 59

McMurray A 1999 *Community Health and Wellness: A Sociologic Approach*. CV Mosby, Sydney

Miracle V 2004 Women and Heart Disease. *Critical Care Nursing* 23(1):53–54

Murray C, Lopez A 1998 *Health Dimensions of Sex and Reproduction*. WHO, Geneva

Novack LL, Novack DR 1996 Being female in the eighties and nineties; Conflicts between new opportunities and traditional expectations among white, middle class, heterosexual college women. *Sex Roles* 35(1/2):57–77

Oswomen 1992 Australia's participation in the UN Declaration on Elimination of Violence Against Women. Office of the Status of Women, Department of the Prime Minister and Cabinet, AGPS, Canberra

Philpot CL, Brooks GR, Lusterman D, Nutt RL 1997 *Bridging Separate Gender Worlds: Why Men and Women Clash and How Therapists Can Bring Them Together*. American Psychological Association, Washington DC

Pretty G 1998 Woman caring for herself. In: Rogers-Clark C, Smith A (eds), *Women's Health: A Primary Health Care Approach*. MacLennan and Petty, Sydney, pp 19–33

Quick A, Wilkinson R 1991 Income and Health. Socialist Health Association, London

Rogers-Clark C 1998 Women and Health, in Rogers-Clark C , Smith A (eds), *Women's Health: A Primary Health Care Approach*, MacLennan and Petty, Sydney, pp 19–33

Steingart RM, Packer M, Hamm P, Colianese ME, Gersch B, Geltman EM 1991 Sex differences in the management of coronary artery disease. *New England Journal of Medicine* 325(4):226–230

Ted W 1995 Physician Contacts by Sex. Men's Web. Online. 25 March 2004 <http://www.menweb.org/throop/health/stat/lifespan.html>

Wenitong M 2001 Indigenous Male Health: A Report for Indigenous Males, Their Families and Communities, and Those Committed to Improving Indigenous Health. Office for Aboriginal and Torres Strait Islander Health (OATSIH), Commonwealth Department of Health and Ageing, Australia

White AK, Cash K 2003 The State of Men: Health Across the 17 European Countries, The European Men's Health Forum. Online. March 23 2004 <www.emhf.org>

Wilson G 1995 *A Phenomenological Approach to Compliance*, Unpublished Masters Dissertation, University of New England, NSW

Woods M 2001 *Killing them subtly—Social determinants in men's health*. Online. 1 March 2004 <http://www.menshealth.uws.edu.au/documents/Which%20men%20are%20sick.html>

World Health Organization (WHO) 2002 WHO Gender Policy: Integrating Gender Perspectives into the Work of WHO. Online. 1 April 2004 <http://www.who.int/gender/mainstreaming/ENGwhole.pdf>

World Health Organization 1998 From Alma–Ata to the Year 2000: Reflections at Midpoint. Geneva, Switzerland, WHO

Wright A 1999 Men's health: What puts men off visiting their GP?. In Proceedings of the 3rd National Men's Health Conference, Alice Springs 5–8 October

Young C 1994 Health and Gender, *Detroit News*, August 30, pp 33–4. In: Cook A 1998 (ed) *Men's Health Concerns Sourcebook*. Omnigraphics, Detroit

# Chapter 5

## Ageing, Health and Illness

*Colleen Cartwright and Victoria Parker*

**This chapter discusses:**

- how and why ageing affects people's lives;
- how the majority of older people live healthy lives in the community;
- the role of health promotion in maintaining healthy ageing;
- the most common health-related challenges experienced by older people;
- the transition to frailty; and
- the role of health professionals when working with older people.

Since 1900, life expectancy at birth in the developed nations of the world has increased steadily (UN World Statistics Pocketbook 2003). This increase in life expectancy has been accompanied by a continuing decline in the mortality rate, mostly because of declining death rates for specific diseases such as cardiovascular disease. Ageing is a global phenomenon; by 2050 the number of older people worldwide is expected to increase from approximately 600 million now to almost 2 billion (Anan 2002).

This chapter will consider the most common health problems experienced by older people; and, in light of the increasing number of older people in Australia, the corresponding need for health care professionals to facilitate the fitness and health of older people. We will also examine the transition from older age into frailty which, while not an inevitable part of ageing, is an area around which a great deal of health care revolves. The story of May will be the focus of this chapter. As you continue to work through this topic, keep May's situation in mind.

## Case Study

May is an older woman (78) living in regional Australia. She lives on her own in a retirement village, and has done so for the past ten years. She has been widowed for thirty years, and has six adult children. Although she has been without a partner for a very long time, she has found tremendous solace in her family and in her friends at the retirement village.

Once her children left home May became involved in voluntary work for the community. She continued to do this for many years, but in her early seventies she decided to give up this work because she found it too taxing. In her sixties and early seventies, May was also heavily involved in caring for her grandchildren. She provided lots of support to her daughters as they struggled to balance work and family, and so May is very close to her ten grandchildren.

Ageing has not always been easy for May. She has osteoarthritis and for the last 20 years this has been steadily worsening. She has always been concerned that some of the physical changes associated with her disorder, along with ageing, would affect her quality of life. Her fears were confirmed when, for example, driving her motor vehicle became difficult as her vision and hearing deteriorated. As she lost her confidence in driving, she was forced to sell her car. She has also developed osteoporosis, and this means she has to take greater care in all she does to avoid broken bones. This loss of independence and curtailing of activity has resulted in May spending less time with her family, especially her grandchildren.

This section will provide an overview of the major physical, social and structural issues affecting the health, wellbeing and independence of older people, and their connection with healthy ageing. These issues include:

- physical and related functional changes associated with normal ageing, and the common psychosocial problems that may result;
- systemic factors such as health promotion and disease prevention programs, in addition to the associated behavioural factors such as exercise and nutrition; and
- attitudinal and quality-of-life factors such as social interaction.

# Changes to health associated with ageing

Despite popular conceptions that view older age in a negative light, it is not an illness. It is 'a life journey to be embraced and celebrated' (Andrews 2002). Increased age and ill health are not synonymous. Although the biomedical model, which conflated old age with illness, has for some time been the dominant paradigm, the reality is that the majority of older people are healthy, active and participate in the community. Studies have confirmed that the current generation of people aged over 70 are healthier and more adaptable than people of the same age ten and twenty years previously (Hermanova 1998). Similarly, more than two-thirds of older Australians rate their health as good, very good or excellent; and people over 75 scored the highest in terms of their mental health (AIHW 1998). Even those older people with chronic illness generally maintain satisfaction with life by adjusting their expectations and daily routines. However, ageing in some people is associated with increasing ill health, and you will need to be aware of some of the factors that contribute to this.

## Living with Illness

A biomedical explanation of ageing is that it is the progressive, generalised impairment of function that results in a slowing of the adaptive responses to stressors, and an increased risk of age-related disease (Davies 1998). There is no one point at which a person becomes 'old'; there are certain biological and physiological changes associated with ageing that mean mortality rates rise throughout life from puberty and that the rate is uniform. So theoretically, ageing actually begins around puberty and occurs across a lifetime.

Let's examine some of the biomedical challenges and solutions that may be associated with the ageing process.

May has arthritis, which is the most common long-term condition reported by people aged 65 and over. Damage to the hip and knee joints from arthritis and from other musculoskeletal conditions has restricted May's mobility and increased her social isolation, which can often lead to depression. The primary health burden of this condition is pain. However, improved technology, pharmacological agents and alternative remedies have resulted in many older people experiencing dramatic improvement in their pain and mobility. There has been a dramatic improvement in quality of life and health outcomes following hip or knee replacement operations for many older Australians.

Many women of May's generation are, like her, also at risk of developing osteoporosis. This condition, roughly translated as 'porous bones', is characterised by deterioration of bone tissue. It is a progressively debilitating disease that results in bone fragility and an increased susceptibility to fracture (Lemone & Bourke 2004). In older people, most fractures occur from a fall and are linked to osteoporosis. Many of these fractures will heal and cause minimal problems; however, others will result in deformity, chronic pain, disability and the need for supportive care.

Vision and hearing impairment are almost as common as arthritis among older Australians (AIHW 1998). For many older people, such impairment is moderate and recent advances in technology now mean that impaired vision and hearing problems are much more amenable to treatment. Vision is more easily corrected with eyeglasses and cataract excission and intraocular lens replacement, and hearing aids are now much more advanced. However, the initial deterioration of sight and hearing can be socially isolating. The very isolating nature of these impairments may mean that the needs of some older people for such treatment can be overlooked. Because May lived alone, for example, her increasing short-sightedness was not noted by her family for some time. Additionally, having a print disability made access to information about government services difficult for her. So the impact of vision and hearing impairment may be underestimated, as it is not as immediately obvious as other impairments. It may not, for example, appear to restrict a person's mobility, but it can have a detrimental effect on communication, social outings, safety and general feelings of self-esteem and self-confidence.

Because of her problems with arthritis and her vision, May can no longer use a vacuum cleaner or clean her house. She is now reliant on community services to drive her to the shops for groceries and to help with her housework. Because of her mobility problems and the pain they cause, May does not go out very much, and is in danger of becoming socially isolated—a situation which frequently leads to depression. It is important for nurses to remain sensitive to these functional impairments and provide assistance and support so older clients avoid injury and are not socially disadvantaged.

Other conditions, such as cardiovascular changes, cancer, diabetes, and adverse drug reactions, are increasingly common as we age. As discussed in Chapter 3, cardiovascular disease (including coronary heart disease and stroke) is the most common cause of death and disability in older people in Australia, the UK and USA, and its risk factors are now well known lifestyle issues (AIHW 2002). There have, however, been improvements in this area in recent years. In Australia, death rates from cardiovascular disease are declining (AIHW 1998).

Due to the cellular processes associated with normal ageing, the older we get, the more likely we are to develop cancer. More than one-third of cancer deaths in Australia occur in people aged 75 years or over (AIHW 1998). The incidence of breast cancer is higher in older women, yet screening mammography, which is believed to detect cancers amenable to treatment, is under-utilised among this group (Scinto et al 2001). For men, the most common cancer, apart from non-melanocytic skin cancer, is prostate cancer. Colorectal cancer is the second most common cancer in males and females.

Another common lifestyle related disease that is increasingly implicated in the death of the older person is diabetes. Although diabetes was ranked seventh in terms of major conditions causing death in people aged 65 years and over in the 1995 National Health Survey, there is an increasing incidence of this disease in the community. In addition, it is a major problem for the Indigenous population, which has one of the highest prevalence rates of type 2 diabetes in the world (AIHW 1998).

Older people often metabolise drugs at a different rate to younger people, and if their prescribing doctor overlooks this point, adverse reactions can occur. Because older people have more chronic illnesses, they are more likely to be taking multiple medications concurrently. This is also known as polypharmacy. Rochon & Gurwitz (1997) urge cautious use of drugs prescribed for older people and suggest that, in many cases such as osteoarthritis, measures such as gentle exercises and weight reduction may be effective alternatives. A risk of drug side-effects is 'the prescribing cascade'. This can occur when an adverse drug reaction is misinterpreted as a new medical condition, and a new drug is prescribed for the 'new' condition, placing the patient at risk of further adverse effects from what is, in reality, unnecessary treatment. May, for example, has had osteoarthritis for past 20 years and it was steadily worsening. At one stage she was taking a 'cocktail' of drugs to deal with her problem, none of which seemed to work. The pain woke her during the night and she began to use sleeping tablets. May was initially resistant to the idea of trying options other than medication to relieve her pain, such as exercise, and stated firmly that 'rest is the answer'.

In terms of intellectual function, crystallised intelligence, that is, such things as knowledge, wisdom and vocabulary, are generally maintained with increasing age. Neuro-psychological testing does show, however, a slowing of central processing time and acquisition of new information, as well as the decline of what is called fluid intelligence. For example, it can become more difficult as we age to sort new information into categories. Slight memory loss is common with ageing, but it is not usually sufficient to cause problems with daily functioning. Within the general community there are older people with some memory impairment, who nevertheless have normal physical and mental functioning. This condition is called mild cognitive impairment (MCI) (Hogan & McKeith 2001) and people with MCI do have an increased risk of developing dementia (see below).

# Preventing ill health in older people

There is evidence to suggest that, with increasing age, environmental factors, behavioural actions and preventive measures in earlier life become more important than genetic factors in determining good health (Hermanova 1998). For this reason, health promotion strategies for older people have focused on health conditions that are potentially preventable or able to be postponed; have a significant bearing on the independence and wellbeing of older people; and have important consequences for the health system and demands on its performance (Teshuva et al 1994). In the foreseeable future, nurses and allied health professionals are likely to occupy an even greater role in health promotion and disease prevention than has been the case in recent times, possibly in conjunction with general practitioners. It is vital that all health professionals working with older people are well prepared to respond to these challenges. There are a number of health promotion strategies that are proven to promote health and prevent disease in older people. These include improving the individual's level of physical activity, their nutritional status, and reducing their smoking and alcohol consumption; all of which may be amenable to health promotion strategies, even among older people.

The benefits of physical activity are well documented. Exercise can help weight control, increase feelings of wellbeing, aid digestion, decrease stress and tension, increase immunity, prevent premature ageing, improve balance, circulation, flexibility of joints, and improve sleep. Physical activity among older people has also been shown to offer some protection against a number of diseases and conditions, including coronary artery disease, stroke, diabetes, and mental disorders (Munro et al 1997). In addition, exercise is a major component of health promotion activities that aim to prevent falls, because exercise improves muscle strength and balance (Lord et al 1997).

## Case study . . . *continued*

Since she sought comprehensive advice about her medical problems, May has been well informed about prevention of symptoms and complications, and self-management of her osteoarthritis. In particular, physical activity and regular low level exercise are recommended as keeping joints mobile improves the cartilage and eases and nourishes painful arthritic structures. May particularly enjoys her water exercise or hydrotherapy program because she can exercise her painful joints without putting them under strain. May has noticed that her six-month participation in the program has increased her muscle strength and flexibility, making life's little challenges somewhat easier. Apart from the physical benefits, May also enjoys the social contact as the program is conducted in the convenience of the retirement village in which she resides.

Balanced nutrition and access to healthy foods are key factors in the health and wellbeing of older people, as they are in all people regardless of age. Poor nutrition can lead to illness and disease, and the reverse is also true; that is, that ill health can result in poor nutrition. Frail older people are most at risk, but poor nutrition in otherwise well community-dwelling older people is also a serious problem. Although concerns about nutrition often focus on risks associated with being overweight, Williams et al (1998) found that one in three Australians over the age of 60 are at high risk, and one in two were at moderate risk of developing diseases related to under nutrition. Dental problems, including badly fitting dentures that affect chewing and digestion, can exacerbate nutritional problems for older people.

Chapter 3 demonstrated that cigarette smoking may cause ill health at any age; however, its effects often become most apparent in older age. Smoking plays a major role in many diseases, including myocardial and cerebral infarction, lung and other cancers, and chronic lung conditions such as chronic obstructive airways disease (AIHW 1998). In addition, the long-term effects of excessive alcohol consumption can be debilitating in older people because of damage to the liver, brain, pancreas, cardiovascular, haematological and gastrointestinal systems and memory. However, light to moderate intake of alcohol can reduce the risk of heart disease (AIHW 1998). While tobacco and excessive alcohol consumption can contribute to adverse long-term health outcomes, fortunately changing negative habits even in older age can produce health benefits.

# Psychosocial aspects of ageing

Growing older inevitably leads to significant life changes with psychosocial as well as physical challenges. This next section considers the psychosocial aspects of some key issues confronting people as they age.

## Community attitudes

Attitudes to ageing, and to older people, can significantly affect the uptake of health promotion strategies, and therefore healthy ageing and quality of life. Many current views about older people are based on out-dated, incorrect and frequently discriminatory viewpoints. Some people in the community, including health professionals, perceive ageing as a period of inevitable decline accompanied by illness, senility and dependence on others (Bevan & Jeeawody 1998). In reality, this will only be true for a small percentage of older people, at least until they reach their late 80s or 90s.

Ageism may often be unconscious and may manifest in how an event is interpreted. For example, if an older person has a fall this may be seen as evidence that the person is frail and needs institutional care. If a younger person falls, it is more likely to be seen as simply an accident. Similarly, an older person who struggles to remember something may be seen as forgetful in a situation where a younger person is seen as having too much on their mind. The media is usually only interested in the 'doom and gloom' and 'victim' stories (McCulloch 1995). In addition, in our youth-centred, body-beautiful society, older men and women not only have to deal with the bodily changes associated with ageing, but also society's negative reaction to those changes. This may affect their confidence to make love with their partners, particularly when the myth still survives that older people are not sexual beings (see also Quality of life, below). However, reverse ageism that tries to deny any of the problems of ageing, or headlines such as '80-year-old woman climbs Mt Everest' may make a normal older person feel as if they are inferior in some way.

Community attitudes to older people, however, are slowly changing. This is due to the inevitable ageing of our population and the increasing recognition of the significant contribution older people make to society, including as carers (both of children and of other older people) and through extensive volunteering service, including in hospitals, day respite centres and home-based community care. However, if ill health means that an older person cannot contribute in this way, they may be at risk of negative attitudes by others. Nurses need to be aware of, and continually monitor, their own reactions and behaviour to ensure that they do not patronise older patients or infringe their right to self-determination.

## Quality of life

The quality of life of older Australians is generally very good, and is certainly better in many respects than that enjoyed by their parents. This is partly due to their improved health and the fact that physical capacities in old age have increased in recent decades (Kendig & Browning 1997). Psychosocial factors that contribute to the maintenance and enhancement of high quality of life in late adulthood include good physical health, financial stability, family dynamics and cohesiveness, social support networks, maintenance of optimal level of cognitive functioning, personal control and prevention of depression (Yoon 1996).

Quality of life in older people is strongly related to their ability to maintain independence and control. However, it may be difficult for older people to maintain control when dealing with the health system and bureaucracies that often fail to recognise their needs, or tend to 'do for' an older person rather than removing barriers to allow them to do for themselves. Families can also fall into this trap and take over tasks an older person is still capable of doing for themselves. This can occur when family members mistakenly believe they are doing the person a service, or because they become impatient when the older person takes longer to perform the task than the younger person does. May experiences this occasionally with the home care help she receives weekly from a young woman from a local care agency, who insists on moving May's favourite chair because she thinks May could trip over it. In fact, because she is used to having the chair where it is, May never trips over it but occasionally the young woman does. May has stopped arguing with the young woman and just waits until she leaves, and then moves the chair back to where she likes it.

Having supportive relationships is an important aspect of quality of life. The vast majority of older people are satisfied with their personal and emotional life (Queensland Dept of Families 2002) and for many this will continue into their older age. Gender issues are important to consider here. Marriage has been found to be beneficial to the health of men but not necessarily of women, who appear to benefit as much or more from relationships with friends and other relatives (Teshuva et al 1994). May has a loving family and good friends, and is financially stable though not wealthy by any reckoning. Certainly her arthritic pain and lack of mobility bother her, but she enjoys spending time with family and friends, and is particularly active on her computer. Having access to the Internet has allowed her to keep in touch with loved ones living away, and she enjoys researching her family tree using Internet resources.

Stereotypes about ageing and sexuality may influence how older people both think and act sexually. This can lead to gross errors in the clinical management of the sexual concerns of older people (LoPiccolo 1991). There is increasing evidence that people 65 years or older not only continue to enjoy sexual activity to the end of their lives (despite taking a little longer to achieve the same result as previously) but that they are often having as much sex as, and in some cases more than, people 18 to 26 (Steinberg et al 1995). While loss of a partner and physical disability may deprive some older people of opportunities to express their sexuality, a natural desire for close personal contact is retained.

## Transition to frailty

Although the majority of people will remain well and continue to live in their own homes as they age, some will progress to a degree of frailty requiring either intensive home-based care (usually only possible where there is a resident carer) or relocation to a residential aged care facility (RACF). The transition to frailty may occur suddenly as the result of an illness, such as stroke, or an injury such as a fractured neck of femur following a fall. On the other hand, an older person may gradually realise that she or he can no longer perform their normal activities of daily living, such as hygiene and meal preparation, without help. This is certainly becoming the case for May.

A time of great risk for the transition to frailty is when an older person is admitted to hospital. However, a hospital admission also provides an excellent opportunity to address risk factors. Elderly patients with acute illnesses frequently present with functional disability. The main areas of concern are 'the four Is': immobility, instability, incontinence, and intellectual (cognitive) impairment. None of these are caused simply by old age. They are the result of abnormal pathological processes and, as far as possible, must be remedied to prevent disability, loss of independence and institutionalisation. It is advisable that rehabilitation and discharge planning begin from the day of admission if a risk assessment indicates one of these four impairments is possible. A multidisciplinary team approach involving nursing, medical and allied health professionals is also essential. If the conditions cannot be remedied, their effects can be ameliorated, thus restoring functional capacity to the patient and restoring independence (Nair & Cartwright 2003). The 'four Is' will now be considered in more detail.

## Living with Illness

### Immobility

Causes of immobility may be physical, emotional, cognitive and/or social. Physical barriers include joint problems, neurological deficit, impaired balance, stroke, Parkinson's disease, impaired vision, impaired proprioception, cardiovascular and respiratory disease, as well as falls and fear of further falls. Older people may also have problems with their feet, which can be a major hindrance to mobility. May's problem with mobility is largely because of pain, especially in the morning. She is conscious of the risk of falling and hence always extremely cautious. Psychological issues also contribute to immobility. These can include reduced expectations of an active life; loss of adaptability and creativity; introversion with reduced social contact; anxiety and fear of going out. Social factors that can lead to immobility may include retirement, with dangers of reduced income and social contact; living alone; insufficient outside interests or activities; and urgency incontinence, leading to fear of social embarrassment.

The consequence of immobility in older people is loss—loss of choice concerning where they want to be or what they want to do; loss of capability, for example, in getting to the toilet in time or answering the door; loss of social responsiveness; and loss of independence. An older person's world may thus contract, eventually to what is sometimes called a triangular existence—from bed to chair to commode. Prevention of immobility begins in middle age and involves the maintenance of physical fitness and adequate diagnosis/treatment of minor ailments before they become major.

### Instability/falls

Approximately 30% of people over 65 experience at least one fall per year. Falls among older people are a major cause of death and disability, and frequently lead to institutionalisation. Many hospital admissions result in the need for (although not necessarily the receipt of) extensive rehabilitation. Although only about 5% of falls result in fractures and 5% in soft tissue injuries, the remaining 90% may result in loss of confidence.

The causes of falls are numerous and more than one factor may contribute to a fall at any one time. Factors include physical issues, such as impaired balance, arthritis, muscle weakness, foot problems, visual impairment and cardiovascular issues; environmental factors, such as lack of grab rails; and neurological factors such as confusion, cerebrovascular disease, Parkinsonism and epilepsy.

Polypharmacy is also a major and potentially modifiable risk factor for falls, particularly among older people in residential care. Those most often associated with falls are antidepressants, antipsychotics, diuretics and benzodiazapines. Chan & Gibian (1994) found that prescribing short half-life instead of long half-life psychoactive drugs significantly reduced falls among older people in residential care. Rehabilitation and a multidisciplinary approach will not only restore confidence but also increase stability and help to ensure safety if falls occur.

### Incontinence

Incontinence of urine affects a significant proportion of the population, with estimates ranging from 5–30 percent of all Australian women. Although incontinence is not restricted to women or to older people like May, women are much more likely to suffer from it and the prevalence increases significantly with age. Incontinence is one of the major factors leading to institutional placement and has obvious sociocultural implications in our society. Although the functional aspects of incontinence are well researched, it is still a hidden problem that people are reluctant to discuss. Incontinence is highly responsive to treatment in many cases. This may be as simple as general education and advice, such as adjusting fluid intake, pelvic floor exercises, or assessing and modifying those medications that exacerbate the problem. May has this problem, along with millions of other Australians. She thought incontinence was inevitable, especially being a woman who gave birth to six children; in fact, she suffered the embarrassment and turmoil for years before she saw an ad on the television offering free advice and support. May has even been a participant in action research with her support group looking at a continence management model for community patients and nurses.

Faecal incontinence is also a problem with distressing psychosocial implications for some older people. The aetiology is usually multifactorial, with the most common cause being faecal impaction, which may include massive faecal loading with soft or even liquid stool. Immobile patients tend to be slow to respond to the 'call to stool'. They are therefore liable to faecal incontinence when they are given a laxative, especially with potent preparations. This should always be remembered when older patients are being prepared for a barium enema, colonoscopy or surgery. Faecal incontinence should be seen as a curable and preventable problem. It must not be accepted as inevitable.

## Cognitive impairment

Cognitive impairment implies a global disturbance of brain function, affecting memory, orientation, attention and logical thought. Cognitive impairment is a syndrome, not a diagnosis. It may also lead to social problems; for example, neglect of appearance or hygiene and withdrawal from social surroundings, and behavioural problems such as wandering or leaving the stove on. Other issues that may arise from cognitive impairment include poor compliance with medication, incontinence, and stress to carers (with potential for abuse). Common causes include dementia, delirium and depression (discussed further, below).

Dementia is not a normal or inevitable part of ageing. Only 6% of people aged 65 and over have some form of dementia (Queensland Dept of Families 2002). However, it is an age-related disorder, and 24% of people aged 85 years and over can be expected to develop some form of dementia. Because the population is ageing, the number of people with dementia is expected to increase substantially over time (Jorm & Henderson 1993). The most common causes of dementia in older people are Alzheimer's disease and vascular dementia. Symptoms of dementia may include memory loss and impaired concentration, impaired comprehension and the gradual loss of ability to undertake the normal tasks of everyday living. Alzheimer's disease typically has a slow onset, steady progression, early memory impairment, and often has a family history. In vascular dementia, there are history and clinical examination features of vascular disease both in the brain and systemically. It is rarely possible to cure or arrest dementia. However, it is important to be

**63**

aware of, and address where possible, exacerbating factors, which include infections, inadvertent medication side effects, and worsening behaviour that causes carer stress.

Any systemic illness can produce delirium in an older person, which may be the result of infection, metabolic disturbance, and/or drug toxicity (Levkoff et al 1992). Sedatives and any drug with anticholinergic activities, such as Parkinsonian drugs, can produce delirium. In clinical practice, the boundary line between dementia and delirium is often blurred. Pre-existing cognitive impairment or dementia is associated with an increased risk of delirium. Studies of delirium suggest that it may be substantially less transient than was previously believed and that only a minority of patients fully recover to their previous level of cognitive function after an episode of delirium.

Depression is one of the few reversible causes of cognitive impairment. It is characterised by low or depressed mood, loss of interest in usual activities and is often accompanied by a range of symptoms. Some are somatic, for example appetite and weight disturbance; others, like May's, are psychological and include difficulty concentrating and negative thoughts. It is not always easy to diagnose and mild depression is frequently missed. May was feeling low for some time before she happened to mention it to her daughters, who urged her to find help. General population studies have shown that approximately 10–20% of older people report significant depressive symptoms. However, this is much less the case for major depressive illness. Generally, except for those older people in residential care, the prevalence of depression is very low (AIHW 1999). It has been suggested that only between 0.5% and 3% of community dwelling older people will experience a major depressive episode (Byrne 1993).

Although not a symptom in itself, one outcome of depression is suicide. Many people are unaware that the highest per capita rate of suicide occurs in older men, particularly those over 80 (AIHW 1998). It is also possible that the rate of suicide generally is seriously under-reported. Many health professionals and community members in Australia continue to believe that suicide is a criminal offence (Steinberg et al 1995), which it has not been in any state/territory of Australia for more than a decade. Such beliefs may result in under-reporting, for fear of legal consequences to the patient (where the suicide was not completed) or their family. As well as affecting data collection, and hence a true understanding of the extent of the problem, it may also mean that a person who has attempted (but not completed) suicide may not receive appropriate counselling and support.

There are a number of inevitable losses that occur with ageing. The concepts of loss and grief are discussed fully in Chapter 10, but it is important to note here that a significant part of the ageing experience also includes the loss of loved ones when friends and family of a similar age die. The loss of a spouse or partner after many years together can be particularly devastating. Dealing with such losses requires substantive coping strategies, which may be diminished by poor health or other stressors such as financial worries. Loss and grief at any age can trigger a depressive episode. It is important that older people receive counselling and support for these losses, and that they not be seen as just a normal part of ageing.

# Personal safety for the older person

A major issue of personal safety for older patients is elder abuse. This may occur in the patient's home or in an institutional setting, such as a hospital or RACF. Elder abuse takes a number of forms, which include psychological abuse (including verbal abuse), physical abuse (including sexual abuse), economic abuse, and both passive and active neglect (James 1992).

Elder abuse is a complex subject, and in a domestic situation the abuser may be in as much need of assistance as the abused person, for example, because of carer burden. Nevertheless, older people have a legal right to protection. Community nurses may become concerned that an older patient is being abused, either directly or through neglect, or may witness institutionalised abuse. As service providers, nurses may have a legal duty of care to report cases of suspected elder abuse. It is important to be familiar with the legislative requirements, as well as services that may be available to support and protect older people who have been, or are at risk of being, abused. In some Australian states/territories it is an offence to fail to bring information about a serious offence to the attention of authorities.

# Discrimination and older people

Older people may experience discrimination in many ways. In terms of health care, this can include care being limited on the basis of age alone. For example, an older person may not have a health problem adequately investigated because the health care provider incorrectly ascribes the condition to the person's age. 'It's just your age, Dear' is not only patronising but may also constitute neglect.

Discrimination may also occur when an older person is treated without their informed consent. Although there is now a much better understanding of the legal requirement of truly informed consent for all patients, this can often be overlooked when treatment is given to an older person. This may be because the nurse or doctor believes (often mistakenly) that the person does not have the capacity to give consent or because older people do not always know their rights and may not complain about such treatment. It is important for nurses and others to understand that if a person is treated without consent, the health care provider may be liable for a charge of assault, even if the treatment given was considered by the health care provider to be in the person's best interest. The only person who can really decide what is in the patient's best interest is the patient themselves, ideally after having discussed the options with a competent health professional. Partly as a consequence of legal arguments, many hospitals today hold pre-operation information sessions some days before scheduled operations, to ensure that patients are fully informed.

A form of discrimination that can be more difficult to detect may occur when an older person is treated with less respect than that shown to younger people. This may extend to such things as: talking down to, or patronising, an older person; calling the person by their given name without their permission, or calling them by a nickname such as Gran or Pop; not

**65**

respecting the privacy, or sexuality, of an older person, including separating couples in RACFs. This last point is less of a problem than it used to be. Such discriminatory practices infringe the ethical principle of the right to equal respect and can seriously affect the health and wellbeing of an older person. It is not difficult to understand how such behaviour could trigger, or exacerbate, depression and loss of self-esteem.

## Advance care planning and older people

Many older people are fearful of what the end stage of their lives will be like and may be concerned about the inappropriate use of technology, especially if they have seen loved ones kept alive by machines beyond the point of any quality of life. In particular, they may be concerned about what will happen when they can no longer speak for themselves. One way of addressing such fears is to assist people to take advantage of legal avenues for advance care planning.

### Case study ... *continued*

May has thought long and hard about death and has very strong views about the 'right to die'. While May still had her autonomy and personal control, she decided to discuss the prospect of dying with her daughters. They agreed to comply with her wishes in the event that something happens and May is left in what she described as a 'vegetable state'. May is fortunate to have had the opportunity to legally document her wishes. Not only has this given her peace of mind but it will also take the burden of such decisions away from her family, unlike some families who agonise over their dying relative. They do not know what decisions to make and experience profound feelings of sadness and guilt as a result.

When working with older clients, an important aspect of care is to introduce the concept of advance care planning while the patient is still healthy. Depending on the legislative options in a specific state or territory, advance care planning options may include the use of written instructions for a future time when the patient has lost capacity (that is, an Advance Health Directive or Living Will) and/or the appointment of a proxy or agent to make decisions at such a time (e.g. under an Enduring Power of Attorney). All states/territories also now have guardianship legislation, under which a person who lacks the capacity to make decisions for themselves can have someone appointed to make decisions for them. Nurses have both a moral and, in some cases, a legal responsibility to ascertain what the current status of legislation is in their own area, and to ask patients if they have made such arrangements.

## Conclusion

This chapter has emphasised that the majority of older people live full and independent lives. Increased age does not necessarily mean ill health; however for some older people physical changes associated with ageing may mean the loss of independent living and related psychosocial issues. As the number of older people increases, there is an urgent need both to maximise wellbeing and to carefully plan to ensure that those who become frail can be cared for appropriately. This planning must incorporate partnerships between all levels of government, increased community awareness and initiatives, health care workforce innovations including training opportunities, and a better understanding of related health problems, some of which require specialised care.

Obviously it is impossible to discuss every issue about ageing in a single book chapter. However this chapter aimed to provide some insight into how ageing and illness affects people's lives and how it is essential that the community, families and especially nurses can strive to promote healthy ageing by encouraging a positive quality of life. There are huge demands on all facets of aged care. These include the standards of our residential care facilities, the morale of aged care workers and carers, and the financial and emotional burden on the families involved. With these challenges in mind, the cultural, economic and social trends of the ageing population mean that our expectations and life style choices are requiring different attitudes.

## Tutorial questions

1. Given your understanding about May, if she was admitted to hospital following a fall, what strategies for her long-term care in the community might you develop during her discharge planning? You will need to consider the physical and psychosocial aspects of her case, such as her level of community and family support, her co-morbidities, and her expressed needs and wishes.

2. Some health care professionals can be rather impatient when providing care to the older patient. Why do you think this happens? How do you think the older person feels if he or she knows they are a hindrance?

3. If you were caring for May during her hospital admission, how might you approach the issue of long-term residential care with her?

## References

Australian Institute of Health & Welfare (AIHW) 1999 *Older Australia at a Glance: Section 15, Healthy Ageing.* Lincoln Gerontology Centre, AGPS, Canberra

—(AIHW) 2002 *Australia's Health 2002.* AIHW, Canberra

—(AIHW) 1998 *Australia's Health 1998.* AIHW, Canberra

Anan K 2002 UN Secretary-General, Address to 2nd UN World Assembly on Ageing, 9th April, Madrid, Spain

Andrews K 2002 Speech presented at the 14th Annual Nursing Issues Congress, 9th May, Sydney

Bevan C, Jeeawody B 1998 *Successful Ageing. Perspectives on Health and Social Construction.* Mosby, Australia

Byrne G 1993 Recognition and Management of Mental Disorders in the Elderly. In: Tippett V, Elvy G, Hardy J, Raphael B *Mental Health in Australia: A Review of Current Activities and Future Directions, Department of Human Services and Health,* AGPS, Canberra

Chan DKY, Gibian T 1994 Medications and Falls in the Elderly. *Australian Journal of Ageing* 13(1):22–26

Davies I 1998 Cellular mechanisms of ageing. In: *Brockelhurst's Textbook of Geriatric Medicine and Gerontology.* Churchill Livingstone, Edinburgh, pp 51–83

Hermanova H 1998 *Multi-Country Perspectives on Healthy Ageing: a Review. Australian Journal of Ageing* 17:1. Special Supplement: World Congress of Gerontology, Adelaide, Australia, 1997

Hogan DB, McKeith I 2001 Of MCI and dementia: Improving diagnosis and treatments. *Neurology* 56:1132

James MP 1992 *The elderly as victims of crime, abuse and neglect.* Trends and Issues 37

Jorm AF, Henderson AS 1993 *The Problem of Dementia in Australia,* 3rd edn, AGPS, Canberra

Kendig H, Browning C 1997 Positive Ageing: facts and opportunities. *Medical Journal of Australia* 167:409

Lemone P, Burke K (eds) 2004 *Medical-Surgical Nursing. Critical Thinking in Client Care,* 3rd edn. Pearson Education Inc, New Jersey

Levkoff SE et al 1992 Delirium—The occurrence and persistence of symptoms among elderly hospitalized patients. *Arch Intern Med* 153:334–340

LoPiccolo J 1991 Counselling and therapy for sexual problems in the elderly. *Clinics in Geriatric Medicine* 7(1):161–179

Lord SR, Ward JA, Williams O, Strudwick M 1997 The Effect of a 12-Month Exercise Trial on Balance, Strength, and Falls in Older Women: A Randomized Controlled Trial. *Journal of the American Geriatric Society* 43:1198–1206

McCullogh S 1995 *Older People and the Law. An Investigation into the Legal and Consumer Needs of Older People in Victoria.* April, Consumer Law Centre Victoria

Moody HR 1996 *Ethics in an Aging Society.* John Hopkins University Press, Baltimore

Munro J, Brazier J, Davey R, Nicholl J 1997 Physical activity for the over-65s: could it be a cost-effective exercise for the NHS? *Journal of Public Health Medicine* 19(4):397–402

Nair B 1999 Older people and medications: what is the right prescription? *Australian Prescriber* 22:130–131

Nair BK, Cartwright CM 2003 Health of older women. In: O'Connor V, Kovacs G (eds) *Obstetrics, Gynaecology and Women's Health,* Cambridge University Press, Melbourne

Pahor M & Applegate WB 1997 Geriatric medicine. *British Medical Journal* 315:1071–1074

Peel N, Cartwright C, Steinberg M 1998 Monitoring slips, trips and falls in the older community: preliminary results. *Health Promotion Journal of Australia* 8(2):148–150

Queensland Department of Families 2002 A*geing: Myth and Reality.* Queensland Government, Brisbane

Rochon PA, Gurwitz JH 1997 Optimising drug treatment for elderly people: the prescribing cascade. *British Medical Journal* 315:1096–1099

Scinto J, Gill TM, Grady JN, Nolmboe ES 2001 Screening Mammography: Is It Suitably Targeted to Older Women Who are Most Likely to Benefit? *Journal of the American Geriatric Society* 49:1101–1104

Steinberg M, Donald K, Clark M, Tynan R 1995 Towards successful ageing in the 21st Century. In: Lupton G, Najman J (eds), *The Sociology of Health and Illness*. Macmillan, Australia

Teshuva K, Stanislavsky Y, Kendig H 1994 *Towards Healthy Ageing*. Collins-Dove, North Blackburn, Victoria.

United Nations 2003 *World Statistics Pocketbook 2003*.United Nations, Geneva

Williams T 1998 Nutrition Issues for Older Aussies. Australian Association of Gerontology, National Newsletter, August, pp 9–10

Yoon G 1996 Psychosocial Factors for Successful Ageing. *Australian Journal of Ageing* 15(2):69–72

# Chapter 6

## Multicultural Issues in Health

*Don Gorman and Odette Best*

**This chapter explores:**
- the significance of the cultural issues that influence health, illness and the provision of health care;
- cultural beliefs in relation to health and wellbeing;
- the principles of cultural safety;
- the health status of Indigenous peoples in Australia; and
- strategies for working in partnership with Indigenous peoples.

This chapter deals with the provision of nursing care to clients from a range of cultural backgrounds. Health beliefs and practices vary from culture to culture, making cultural sensitivity essential to the delivery of effective nursing care. Studies have shown the need for greater knowledge and understanding of cultural differences to enable clinicians to respond more effectively to clients from non-English speaking backgrounds (DiCicco-Bloom & Cohen 2003, Gebru & Willman 2003, Spence 2001). This chapter, then, will look at the significance of culture and how it affects our interactions with others; cultural issues that influence health and health care; and the concept of cultural safety. While it is important that we avoid stereotyping people, examples will be given of some of the common differences in views held by different cultures that demonstrate how cultural differences can affect health care.

While this chapter discusses primarily ethnic cultural groups, it should be borne in mind throughout that other subgroups within society also have their own specific cultural beliefs. They can therefore be disadvantaged if their beliefs differ from mainstream culture. A particular focus of this chapter will be the health needs of Indigenous Australians, a recognised subgroup of Australians, through an exploration of the case study of Irene.

# Case study

Irene is an Indigenous Australian woman in her early thirties from a small rural town. She was diagnosed with chronic renal failure and had to receive treatment for this in a metropolitan renal centre. While in the city, she also had to receive training for self-management of dialysis so she could care for herself when she returned home. In total, her treatment and dialysis training meant Irene spent seven months away from her predominantly Indigenous community, within a health care culture that was quite alien to her:

> 'I had to leave my job and my family and all my friends to come down here. I was scared you know. I'd never been away for so long from my country, and I'd never been away by myself either. I was very lonely. When I wasn't training or being treated at the unit I didn't know where to go or what to do, and I didn't know anyone in that city. Also I'd never really been sick before so I didn't understand half of what the doctors and nurses were saying to me. I preferred to ask the other black fellas in the renal unit. I learned more off my own people about dialysis and what I had to do to manage it than I did from anybody else. There were a lot of them there and we helped each other. The white nurses were good, but they were so rushed all the time.'

# Culture

Irene's story demonstrates that while a great deal has been written about culture, the concept is not well understood outside the discipline of sociology, yet its influence is pervasive. Nurses may be unaware of their own culture or the degree to which their cultural influences affect the way they view people or how they expect them to act in various situations. Culture influences what we expect of our patients as well as what we expect of ourselves as nurses.

Despite its covertness, culture plays a significant part in determining behaviour and influences our knowledge, beliefs, morals, and customs. There are literally thousands of rules that we learn from early childhood to live by, such as when to look someone in the eye and when to look away. Although we are not necessarily conscious of these rules, when someone breaks them, we tend to feel uncomfortable with them. Samovar & Porter (2003, p 8) define these cultural rules as:

> The deposit of knowledge, experience, beliefs, values, attitudes, meanings, social hierarchies, religion, notions of time, roles, spatial relationships, concepts of the universe, and material objects and possessions acquired by a group of people in the course of generations through individual and group striving.

Culture is the worldview of members of the cultural group that sustains it. The most commonly discussed group in the context of multiculturalism is the ethnic group, such as the Indigenous community in which Irene lived. However, a cultural group may also be any cluster of people with a common set of beliefs and values; for example, those based on sexual preferences, age, or gender. Nursing can also be considered a cultural group, with its particular values and beliefs, which distinguish it from other health care professions, and with members who identify with each other as nurses.

While some aspects of culture are acquired through education, much of it is learned unconsciously through contact with other members of the society or group, and especially through childhood experiences with family, friends and school. As cultural values and beliefs tend to be learned unconsciously, the expectations that individuals place on other peoples' behaviour are ingrained and equally unconscious. Irene, for instance, expected her nurses to understand that she needed to learn about her treatments at a different pace and in a different way to Anglo-Celtic people. Similarly, her nurses expected that the way they traditionally taught self-management of dialysis to non-Indigenous people would suffice for an Indigenous woman like Irene. As a result, when the behavioural expectations of people are not met, the reaction of the individual tends to be emotional, automatic, and judgmental. The example given earlier about eye contact is a good case in point. In Anglo-Celtic cultures, there is an expectation that people will look each other in the eye when speaking to them. If this doesn't happen, there is a tendency to suspect that the person is being dishonest based on the assumption that 'one can't look someone in the eye and lie'. Many other cultures however, including many Indigenous Australian communities, consider it rude, disrespectful or even aggressive to look someone directly in the eye, so when people with these different cultural values meet both are likely to feel uncomfortable with the other.

While the existence of culture is universal, all groups tend to have a specific view of the world, and that worldview can vary a great deal between cultures. This fact is one that few individuals are instinctively aware of. Because of the unconscious nature of cultural learning, group values and beliefs tend to be seen as universal; that is, not specific to the individual's own culture. Hence when people from other cultures are met, there is no recognition of the fact that their behaviour is determined by a different set of equally valid rules. Their behaviour is in fact judged unconsciously by the cultural rules of the observer.

Dyer (1997) argues that this occurs because members of the dominant race or culture in any community or society are exempt from being classified by their racial or cultural background. They rarely consider their distinct cultural or racial characteristics because they see themselves as normal. It is members of so-called minority groups who are seen as different. The nurses and the doctors caring for Irene, immersed in the culture of the renal unit, expected her to know instinctively what their medical jargon meant, and what their complex procedures entailed. The situation is akin to an umpire in a football match attempting to apply the rules of cricket to the players and refusing to acknowledge that those rules are game specific rather than universal. This tendency, called ethnocentricity, is a major barrier to cross-cultural understanding.

One of the aspects of behaviour that is determined by culture is that of the roles individuals fulfil and the ways in which they develop and maintain interpersonal relationships. People's place in society, how they interact with each other, and their rights and responsibilities are all determined by their culture. The role of nurses within the health system, for example, is strongly influenced by cultural beliefs about the importance of caring for those who are ill. How we interact with members of other health professions is also influenced by culture. For example, western society highly values medical knowledge and practice, and this means that members of the medical profession are expected to take a leadership role in the health care team, with nurses participating as members of the team.

An individual's values, which are the basis of judgments that they make to determine whether they perceive something as good, bad, desirable or undesirable, are also culturally determined. These values, while often unconscious, play a major role in deciding what behaviours are acceptable and what are not. Society develops rules from these values, which in turn determine behaviour that is rewarded if it complies with the rules, or punished if it does not. To disobey a culture's rules of behaviour invokes a judgment and usually a negative emotional response by members of that culture, often without awareness of the values underlying it, and rarely is there recognition that those values are culture specific. Values also affect the individual's perceptions of others, so that once a person has transgressed a cultural rule, there is a tendency to develop an overall view of that person as deviant, leading to a biased judgment of any future behaviour.

Another aspect of culture is that of symbolism. Over time, all societies develop symbolism in which concepts become value-laden. Symbols developed in past times represent deep-seated values that are rarely understood by the present members of the society. Because these symbols are covert, there is a tendency to assume that they mean the same to everyone regardless of cultural background. This mistaken belief makes cross-cultural understanding especially difficult. A powerful symbol in Anglo-Celtic cultures is that of Christmas. The origin of this symbol is in Christian religion, but most Anglo-Celtic Australians, even those who do not consider themselves to be practising Christians, would consider it unthinkable that they should be expected to work on Christmas Day and not spend it at home with their family.

Within a multicultural society, such as that found in Australia, there are many groups of people who come from non Anglo-Celtic cultural backgrounds. Members of these groups share a common culture, to the extent at least that they have more in common with each other than they have with members of other groups or with the dominant Anglo-Celtic group. While members of a group have much in common, like all members of all cultures, there are individual differences and considerable variation can occur within a society. People from a particular group may have had very different experiences and/or backgrounds. Over time they will also be influenced by their interaction with the dominant culture, as well as other groups that they come in contact with.

Despite these variations within an ethnic group, there are still common values and beliefs that vary from other cultures, and in a multicultural society there is a need for people from different cultures to meet and function together for the benefit of all. It is in this meeting that covert cultural values, beliefs, rules, behaviours and symbols create barriers to understanding and acceptance. There are a number of factors that influence the health of people from cultural minority groups. Being a member of a minority group itself affects health, because perceptions of health are culturally determined and cultural and linguistic factors affect the use of services.

# Being a member of a minority culture

Despite the fact that most migrants have a high standard of health due to immigration requirements, minority groups are commonly disadvantaged in society and this is almost certainly true of cultural groups. Whether the minority group is Indigenous or has migrated to the host country, there is a potential impact on health.

For example, migrants to a country also experience some of the cultural and linguistic barriers to utilising a different health care system. The experience of migration can itself negatively influence their health. For example, there is often a reduction in their socioeconomic status, with even highly qualified professionals commonly not having their qualifications recognised and having to take on unskilled work in their adopted country. They can also experience a major reduction in their support systems due to leaving family, friends, careers, and familiar government/social institutions behind. If they move to a country where the language is different to their first language, they can have the added difficulty of communication hindering their access and participation in health care services. Compounding the above, many immigrants experience culture shock, discrimination and racism. Similarly, as Irene's case demonstrates, minority Indigenous groups experience cultural and linguistic barriers within the Australian health system.

# Culture, health and health care

The host country's health care system will be based in that country's culture. Australia's system, for example, is based on Anglo-Celtic cultural beliefs about health, health-related behaviours and health care. As a consequence, there are enormous cultural differences in the perceptions of health and illness, as well as of health care services including:

- Beliefs about external forces—for example, the effects of things like the weather, spirits or supernatural forces, karma, or luck.
- Individuality—as in the extent to which the person is different from their reference group, or the extent to which the individual defers to the wishes of family members when receiving health care.
- The significance of emotions, which can be seen as causing illness or of being symptomatic, that is caused by the illness.
- The role of the family—ranging from not wanting the family to be involved at all, to expecting that the family or the head of the family make all decisions about care and treatment. Aspects of Irene's Indigenous culture, for example, may mean that it is appropriate for her to consult widely within her kinship system before making treatment decisions.

The concept of multiculturalism emphasises the need to recognise and appreciate the different cultures within a society, considering all to be of equal value. This is a good place to start when working with people from cultures different to one's own, but it may not be enough. Multiculturalism has been criticised because it ignores power differentials between ethnic groups, which are 'manifested ultimately in racism' (Polaschek 1998, p 453). This is particularly relevant when considering the health and wellbeing of Indigenous peoples. Respecting Indigenous cultural beliefs and practices is an essential component of offering holistic nursing care, but hardly enough. As you read through this chapter, you will come to understand that understanding the social position of Indigenous peoples is necessary in order to understand a broad range of Indigenous health issues.

The inter-relationship between health, culture and health care is vividly illustrated by Irene and her people, and is worthwhile exploring at some length here to demonstrate these points. Indigenous health within Australia has received attention both nationally and internationally for some years. Within the last decade, there has been much criticism that mainstream health care facilities are, by and large, inappropriate for the Indigenous people accessing them. There has, however, been increasing acceptance that perhaps this is not only due to the inappropriateness of the mainstream health care system but also the marked differences in the construct of health between Indigenous and non-Indigenous peoples.

In Irene's case, her chronic renal disease is a well-documented result of the westernisation of Indigenous health and the devaluing of Indigenous cultural norms. Indigenous Australians were, at the time of colonisation, a fit and healthy race of people. The Indigenous oral tradition of passing on history, and descriptions by early colonists, relate that the traditional lifestyle was based upon physical exercise that took many forms—hunting and gathering, preparation of food, and also ceremonial activities. As Bartlett (1995) noted, the infectious diseases that were later to decimate Indigenous peoples (such as measles, flu and smallpox) were not present prior to colonisation. The so-called 'lifestyle' diseases, including diabetes, chronic renal failure and heart disease, simply did not occur amongst Indigenous peoples. Whilst Aboriginal health was not perfect, the style of living was more in tune with the environment in which people lived. Diets were good. Bush tucker was plentiful. People lived on their country and accepted the responsibility of caring for their country—protecting water holes and sacred sites. People lived in harmony with their environment, accessing the land resources in a way that protected that resource. Waste disposal was not the major health issue that it is today, partly because of the nomadic lifestyle, and partly because of the lack of consumerism with its non-biodegradable products.

Now, however, Indigenous men and women have a much shorter lifespan than non-Indigenous Australians. In the late 1990s, the life expectancy for an Indigenous male at birth was 56 years. An Indigenous female, in the same period, could expect to live 63 years (ABS 2001). The comparative difference in life expectancy is 20 years between Indigenous males and their non-Indigenous counterparts, and 19 years for females. This substantial difference is all the more distressing when the following is taken into account (Neill 2002, p 11): since 1981, overall life expectancies have shown a marked improvement. This means that the relative mortality gap between black and white Australians has widened during a period when governments were supposedly acting on the principle of Aboriginal self-determination.

Statistics are important indicators, but for Indigenous people health status is not merely the breakdown of facts and figures. The statistical approach is derived from the western medical model, which is not compatible with the Indigenous perspective of health. Within the Indigenous context of health, the biological cannot be separated from the psychological, spiritual and community aspects of health. Indigenous definitions of health reflect this in a way that statistical evidence cannot. This point was eloquently raised by Indigenous peoples nearly a decade ago (ATSIC 1995, p 99):

> A certain kind of industrial deafness has developed. The meaning of these figures is not heard or felt. The statistics of infant and perinatal mortality are our babies and children who die in our arms . . . The statistics of shortened life expectancy are our mothers and fathers, uncles, aunts and elders who live diminished lives and die before their gifts of knowledge and experiences are passed on. We die silently under these statistics.

To Aboriginal people, and to many other ethnic groups, 'health' is much more than the absence of disease and incapacity. It is a matter of determining all aspects of their life, including control over the physical environment, of dignity, of community self-esteem, and of justice. In a similar vein, health care is not merely a matter of the provision of doctors, hospitals, and medicines (National Aboriginal Health Strategy, Working Party 1989, p ix).

In multicultural countries like Australia, government policies emphasise equity for all ethnic groups, but many services do not have staff conversant in their clients' languages or who understand their needs. Irene's case is a typical example. As a result, clients of health care can be seriously disadvantaged in terms of their rights, particularly with regard to informed consent. Lack of information about treatment has been identified as being a major disadvantage of non Anglo-Celtic patients in Australia (Comino et al 2001). Poor communication between health care providers and non Anglo-Celtic clients can result in:

- the client's lack of knowledge of the purpose or side effects of drugs;
- admission to hospital without knowledge of the treatment to be given;
- treatment without consent;
- misidentification of patients;
- inappropriate discharge from hospital; and
- culturally inappropriate treatment; for example, the administration of a blood transfusion to a patient whose religious beliefs forbid it, or the administration of oral medications which contain alcohol to a patient whose culture forbids the intake of alcohol.

# Transcultural perceptions and practices relating to illness and suffering

Responding to the suffering of clients, families, and communities is a central aspect of nursing care. Perceptions, meanings, significance, interpretations, and experiences of suffering vary within cultural groups. Nurses should always be aware that the suffering of their patients is constructed by the individual, their family and community, within their specific sociocultural context.

A person's experience of suffering derives its meaning and significance from the sociocultural context in which it occurs. Culture determines whether they should expect and tolerate suffering in a given situation, and how to behave. Chapter 9 considers the pain and fatigue experience. It's important here to note how culture can influence this experience. For example, women from some cultures are likely to perceive labour pain as an experience of suffering, and react accordingly. Others, by contrast, are more likely to see it as a normal. Members of some cultures, even when they experience pain, are likely to consider it inappropriate to express it. Others simply don't know how to express it in a way that is compatible with the dominant culture.

While the way pain is expressed is culturally determined, it is also responded to in culturally prescribed ways. In other words, responses entail culturally specific and symbolic (often ritualised) caring actions, so that the judgments and interpretations by nurses to other people's suffering is also a cultural interpretation. For example, Anglo-Celtic cultures tend to endorse the attitude of stiff upper lip. That is, it is expected that the expression of suffering will be minimal, and the person who overtly expresses pain may be considered weak, cowardly, or attention seeking. Anglo-Celtic nurses therefore may well judge clients who come from cultures that openly express suffering as not deserving of attention, and even be reluctant to respond to patients' complaints.

Personal beliefs and values about, and attitudes towards, what is suffering, the meaning of suffering, what constitutes suffering and how it is communicated will influence a nurse's judgments, as well as how they interact with patients.

Only by asking people to interpret their behaviour can nurses infer whether someone is suffering or not. There is, however, always a risk that they will interpret other people's suffering from their *own* point of view or perspective, rather than the patient's. Irene, for example, responded to her emotional pain at being separated from her kin and country in silence— which many Anglo-Celtic nurses who care for Indigenous Australians may interpret as stoicism or compliance rather than the sadness and loneliness that she actually felt.

Anglo-Celtic health care claims it is based on objective scientific knowledge. Treatment is grounded in scientifically proven data about cause and effect. This strengthens the ethnocentric tendency to believe that the care is unquestionably correct and will therefore succeed. However, there is another factor that is extremely important in the success of all treatment—the patient believing in the treatment. This factor, known as the placebo effect, is stimulated by cultural rituals, communication processes, trust and faith in the carer and healing practices (Helman 1994). If the client does not believe in the treatment, regardless of its scientific basis, not only is it less likely to be effective, but they are also less likely to participate in it.

# Examples of cultural health beliefs

While it is important not to stereotype according to cultural background, the following are some common examples of perceptions and attitudes towards health and health care that are not generally held in Anglo-Celtic cultures. Health may be attributed to good luck or to leading a good life, either in the past or the present, or to the balance of yin and yang.[1] 'Hot' and 'cold'[2] are often substituted for yin and yang. Health can also be a result of purification rituals such as hot spring baths and herbal infusions. Ill health, on the other hand, can be caused by evil spirits or exposure to polluting sources; such as blood, sick people, and dead bodies. It can also be a result of possession by a demon, the 'evil eye', bad water,[3] possession by ghosts, or other acts of sorcery.

Illness may be treated by Tiger Balm, a mentholated ointment, for a variety of conditions including colds, upset stomach, bruises, and insect bites; tonics, such as ginseng; or coin rubbing[4]. In some cultures, a cloth wrapped around the abdomen provides protection, especially for children, aged, and pregnant women. Moreover, practices that Anglo-Celtic peoples call 'alternative medicine', such as herbalism, acupuncture, moxibustion,[5] Ayurvedic medicine,[6] and cupping[7] are actually mainstream practices in other cultures.

---

[1] Yin and yang: These permeate all of nature. Yang represents activity, the sun, the sunny side of the mountain or river bank, light, warmth and fullness, and hence in traditional Chinese society the dynamic masculine principle. Yin represents substance, the shady side of the mountain or river bank; darkness, coldness and emptiness, the receptive feminine principle.

[2] Hot and cold: Foods are classified on a continuum as hot, warm, neutral, cool or cold. This is not in terms of temperature or spiciness but reflects their level of action on the metabolism. If a person complains of being 'hot', their metabolism is running at a faster rate and the core temperature will be slightly elevated. This will be associated with feeling hot, wearing less clothes than others and being more hungry, thirsty and restless, with tendencies toward constipation, dark urine and hoarseness. All medicines are classified in the same way (heteropathic medicine); hot herbs will be used for a cold disease pattern and so forth.

[3] Wind (or air) and water: Are seen as the carriers of perverse influences into the body. Wind causes headaches, trembling and paralysis. Wind cold causes aches, pains, chills and fevers while wind heat causes sore throats and high fevers. 'Bad' water will act first on the GI tract then produce more chronic conditions.

[4] Coining or spooning: Scraping the skin with a spoon or coin to dramatically stimulate circulation and a localised immune reaction. Will often leave red abraded areas and bruises.

[5] Moxibustion: The burning of small balls of moxa or dried mugwort (*Artemesia vulgaris*) directly on appropriate acupuncture points. The moxa may also be placed on a slice of ginger or garlic or slid over the end of an in-place acupuncture needle. This produces a very intense infra red exposure to that area with resultant pain reduction and myofascial release.

Aboriginal communities such as Irene's also have their own traditional medicinal practices that have been effectively administered and valued for generations. Unfortunately, as part of the colonisation process, these treatments and practices were superseded by western medical practices. This happened even though traditional Indigenous practices were tested within western means, and were often deemed effective. For example, Lawson Holman found confirmation of the effectiveness of a particular traditional treatment. Patients with lacerations and compound fractures occasionally arrived at the hospital with 'antbed' plasters on their wounds, made from material obtained from specific types of anthills. These were usually promptly replaced with a conventional dressing. Having noticed that there seemed to be more problems with infection following removal, Holman opted in certain cases to leave the antbed plaster on, with good results. Subsequent testing demonstrated antimicrobial properties (Hunter 1993, p 55).

Health problems, such as the high incidence of renal failure in Irene's people, are largely attributed to the fact that prior to the establishment of Aboriginal Medical Services in the early 1970s, Aboriginal health was administered under western management theories (the provision of hospitals and doctors), which originated in English-speaking countries such as the United States and Britain. The decline of Indigenous health is also indicative of the inappropriateness of this model. Australian Indigenous peoples, and other ethnic minority groups, have therefore found the Anglocentric health care system to be at times unbending, culturally inappropriate, difficult to understand and alienating.

# Conclusion—How do we work with people from different cultures?

This chapter has demonstrated that nursing has a culture of its own that is based in the values and beliefs of mainstream culture. It is important for any health professional to realise that their caring beliefs and practices are not *universal*. It is critical that we care for people in a way that is appropriate to the client's cultural background. To achieve this, nurses need to be educationally prepared to address the many complex problems associated with working with people from different cultures. In addition, we should be aware of the power imbalance between the culturally dominant health provider and the culturally subordinate health client and strive to provide culturally safe care. Clients from most non-Anglo-Celtic cultures can feel overawed by the Australian health care system and the nurses who work within it, seeing them as highly knowledgeable and powerful. They may also be anxious or afraid, hence will be reluctant to question authority or believe they must do whatever they are told. It is important to be aware of this and make an effort

---

[6] Ayurvedic medicine: The ancient Indian medical system.

[7] Cupping: Placing a hot cup on the body and letting it cool until the air contracts and draws the skin upward. Professional cupping is usually done with a small suction pump attached to the cup. Cupping causes localised hydration and myofascial release. Bruising may occur in some people.

to empower clients, encouraging them to express their opinions and request that their values and beliefs are taken into consideration.

It is also important for nurses to understand the criticisms that have been levelled against the nursing profession in relation to its capacity to respond to the needs of people from non-dominant cultures. One critique which has received a lot of recent interest is Puzan's (2003) claim that the nursing culture is marked by its white cultural dominance. In her paper, 'The Unbearable Whiteness of Being (In Nursing)', she explains what 'whiteness' means (p 195):

> One of the markers of white privilege is its authority; its ability to stipulate and validate the rules and regulations of everyday concourse and discourse. In this manner, whiteness determines what counts as knowledge, membership, and language.

This 'whiteness' of nursing means that people who are different to the mainstream (for example, from an ethnic background which is not Anglo-Celtic) may feel out of place if they attempt to join the profession, because nursing is so strongly influenced by 'white' culture. This is of concern because nursing as a profession benefits when people from many different cultural backgrounds choose to become nurses, as this increases the capacity of nursing to provide culturally appropriate care to different groups of people.

Furthermore, Puzan argues that nurses expect their patients to 'conform to and comply with the norms of standardized care, ignoring not only racial, but gender and class differences as well' (2003, p 197). Patients who do not conform may be at risk of being negatively judged, which could then influence the quality of nursing care provided to them. For example, the Indigenous woman who chooses to have her baby on her homeland rather than in hospital may be seen as a poor mother who has jeopardised the health of her baby as well as herself. That it might be important for this woman that her baby is born on her homeland may not be understood (Kildea 1999).

In response, the concept of cultural safety was developed in New Zealand by Maori nurses who sought to analyse nursing practice from their perspective as members of an Indigenous minority group. It is seen as an ethical standard which commences with a recognition of the position of certain groups within a society (Polaschek 1998). As such it is an important starting point for nurses who seek to provide high quality care to their patients.

Culturally safe care is the effective care of a person or family from another culture by a practitioner who has undertaken a process of reflection on their own cultural identity, and who recognises the impact of their own culture on their practice. Unsafe cultural practice is any action that diminishes, demeans or disempowers the cultural identity and wellbeing of an individual (Adapted from the New Zealand Nursing Council *Guidelines for Cultural Safety in Nursing and Midwifery Education*, Nursing Council of New Zealand 2003). The key to culturally safe practice lies in becoming aware of one's own cultural values and beliefs; a realisation that these are not universal; and that to provide appropriate care it is necessary to explore the client's values and beliefs with them to ensure that care is congruent with the client's culture. To do otherwise is to make the client culturally unsafe.

Ramsden (1992) identified cultural safety as best practice for nurses in caring for peoples from differing cultures. Ramsden argued that people feel culturally safe when they perceive that they are recognised within the health care system and are assured that the system reflects something of them—their culture, language, customs, attitudes, beliefs and preferred ways of doing things. For nurses, this is difficult because of the portrayal of Indigenous Australians so pervasive in all forms of media. Too often we see images of violence, unemployment and drug and alcohol abuse among differing Indigenous communities. This can lead to a perception that all Indigenous Australians struggle with these issues, which is simply not the case.

This perception can have disastrous consequences. For instance, several years ago in an Indigenous community there was yet another black death in custody. A young Indigenous man was found unconscious in a park where Indigenous peoples often went to consume alcohol. When the police took him into custody for being drunk and disorderly, it was assumed that he was drunk as he smelt of alcohol, and so he was placed in a lock up to sleep it off. Unfortunately this young man was not under the influence of any substance but was a diabetic, and had fallen into a diabetic coma. The result of this faulty diagnosis was that the young man lost his life. This is a tragic consequence of stereotyping.

The question remains about how best to work with Indigenous and other cultural groups, to ensure that health care interventions are appropriate and effective. Nurses will find that the principles of cultural safety will serve them well when working with other cultures. Successful Aboriginal and other cultural health services work from a premise of community ownership, whereby cultural groups make their own decisions about the sorts of health care they need and want for their communities. The nurse who works within these principles, and who genuinely demonstrates respect for other cultures, will be well received and has the potential to contribute significantly to the health and wellbeing of other people.

---

# Tutorial questions

1.  A good place for any health professional to start, when considering their practice in relation to people from cultures different from their own, is to reflect on their cultural beliefs. You can do this by considering how your own health and other beliefs relate to some of the worldviews described in this chapter.

    Choose one ethnic, or other cultural group with which you have come in contact, and consider the following questions:

    a)  How do you feel about those people as a group? Do you have positive or negative perceptions about members of the group, or the group as a whole?

    b)  How did you develop your particular attitudes and beliefs in relation to that group?

    c)  What role has the media played in developing your perceptions of these people?

# References

ATSIC 1995 Second Report. Aboriginal and Torres Strait Islander Social Justice Commissioner, Canberra

Australian Bureau of Statistics 2001 *The Health and Welfare of Australia's Aboriginal and Torres Strait Islander Peoples*. ABS, Canberra

Bartlett B 1995 *An Aboriginal Health Worker's Guide to Family, Community and Public Health*. Central Australian Aboriginal Congress Publication, Alice Springs

Couzos S, Murray R 1999 *Aboriginal Primary Health Care: An Evidence Based Approach*. Oxford University Press, Melbourne

Comino E, Silove D, Manicavasagar V, Harris E, Harris M 2001 Agreement in symptoms of anxiety and depression between patients and GPs: the influence of ethnicity. *Family Practice* 18:71–77

DiCicco-Bloom B, Cohen D 2003 Home Care Nurses: A Study of the Occurrence of Culturally Competent Care. *Journal of Transcultural Nursing* 14:25–31

Dyer R 1997 *White*. Routledge, New York

Gebru K, Willman A 2003 A Research-Based Didactic Model for Education to Promote Culturally Competent Nursing Care in Sweden. *Journal of Transcultural Nursing* 14:55–61

Helman C 1994 *Culture Health and Illness*, 3rd edn. Butterworth Heinemann, Oxford

Hunter E 1993 Aboriginal Health and History: Power and Prejudice in Remote Australia. Cambridge Press, Hong Kong

Kildea S 1999 *And the women said . . . reporting on birthing services for Aboriginal women from remote top end communities*. Women's Health Strategy Unit, Territory Health Services, Darwin

National Aboriginal Health Strategy (NAHS) Working Party 1989, National Aboriginal Health Strategy Working Party Report. AGPS Canberra

Neill R 2002 *White out: How Politics is Killing Black Australia*. Allen & Unwin, Crows Nest

Nursing Council of New Zealand 2003, Guidelines for cultural safety, the Treaty of Waitangi, and Maori health in nursing and midwifery education and practice. Online. 30 June 2003, 2003, from <http://www.nursingcouncil.org.nz/culturalsafety.pdf>

Polaschek NR 1998 Cultural safety: a new concept in nursing people of different ethnicities. *Journal of Advanced Nursing* 27:452–457

Puzan E 2003 The unbearable whiteness of being (in nursing). *Nursing Inquiry* 10(3):193–200

Ramsden I 1992 *Kawa Whakaruruhau: Guidelines for Nursing and Midwifery Education*. Nursing Council of New Zealand, Wellington, New Zealand

Samovar L, Porter R 2003 *Intercultural communication: A reader*, 10th edn, Wadsworth, Australia

Spence D 2001 Prejudice, Paradox, and Possibility: Nursing People From Cultures Other Than One's Own. *Journal of Transcultural Nursing* 12:100–106

# Chapter 7

## Health Issues for People in Rural and Remote Areas

*Cath Rogers-Clark and Alexandra McCarthy*

**This chapter examines:**

- definitions of 'rural';
- the incidence of chronic illness and mental illness in rural and remote Australia;
- issues surrounding the delivery of rural health care for those experiencing illness; and
- the role of rural nurses.

In this large land, it will not surprise you to learn that people living outside metropolitan areas often experience life in quite different ways from city dwellers. The vast distances in rural Australia, plus the differences in living conditions, lifestyle and culture between city and country mean that health care for rural people needs to be considered within the context of rural life. That is, nurses and other health care professionals need to learn much more about rural life and rural communities, and appreciate the particular difficulties that confront rural people dealing with health problems, as well as the benefits of rural living and rural communities that help people get through difficult times.

In this chapter, we will explore these issues by considering the Brown family's experiences with illness.

## The Brown family

Louise and her husband Bob, both aged in their sixties, worked and lived on a farm which had been passed down to Louise by her parents. Bob had grown up on a nearby farm, and so he had a wealth of experience in working the land, as did Louise. Louise and Bob had three grown children, two girls in their thirties and a son, Des, who was 23. Des still lived at home, and helped them to work the farm, but the two girls had moved to the city and were both settled there now. Louise and Bob were starting to think about taking life a little easier. It had been decided that Des would take over the farm at some stage in the future, and they looked forward to supporting him in this. Financially, though, things were not looking good, with the farm being hit by the worst drought in living memory for the past eight years. Also, the family was just starting to recover from the trauma which occurred when Louise was diagnosed with breast cancer.

Louise spoke to one of the nurses at the hospital about the treatment choices she had made.

## Case study

I decided to have a mastectomy[1] for my breast cancer. I couldn't afford the time or the money to go to the city for eight weeks for radiation treatment, which is what you have to do when you have a lumpectomy.[2] We were in the middle of another drought, and I had just got a job that would help make ends meet. It's bad enough, having to go to the specialist every three months for a check-up. It costs heaps in petrol and time off work, so I needed to keep that job. And we don't get much help from the government for any of my treatment. Anyway, I didn't want to be down there (in the city) on my own.

And you know I reckon you can heal better with the people you know around you. I can handle things better when I'm at home. It's peaceful for me to be in the bush and that's what I mean by healing. Come back to where you're familiar and your mind hopefully gets back to where it used to be . . . I'm sort of born to be a bushie. I feel very closed up in the city.

I just wish I could get down to see my specialist in the city soon though . . . but I can't get away until we've finished harvesting. To be honest with you, I'm a bit worried with the swelling in my arm, and it would be good to have someone who really knows what they're talking about to tell me whether the cancer has come back or not. I haven't told anyone here I'm worried but, you know, it never sort of leaves you, the worrying.

## What is 'rural'?

It is important to define what we mean by 'rural' before we talk about the issues that can affect the experience of illness for people who live in the country, like Louise and her family. This is because definitions of rural have important implications for the way health services are provided throughout Australia, and the range of services that are available to cancer survivors

---

[1] A mastectomy involves removal of the cancerous breast.

[2] A lumpectomy is surgical removal of the cancerous lump plus some of the surounding tissue but not the whole breast.

and other people with chronic illnesses. Rural Australia also has distinct geographical, cultural and social characteristics that influence the health and psychosocial wellbeing of the people who live there, and the ability to provide health and other services consistent with their needs (Coakes & Kelly 1997).

Around one-third of Australians live away from major cities (Australian Institute of Health and Welfare 2003). Although many attempts have been made, it is not easy to define rural communities (Reid & Solomon 1992). It is well recognised, however, that rural Australians are geographically isolated because of the vast distances and dispersed populations which are a feature of rural Australia. For this reason, there are currently two definitions frequently used in Australia.

The most common definition is the Rural, Remote, Metropolitan Areas Classification (RRMAC) developed by the Department of Primary Industries and Energy (Department of Primary Industries and Energy 1991). The RRMAC uses a combination of population size, distance from major services or towns and population density to categorise communities (Reid & Solomon 1992). For example, some communities are a long way from the nearest city in terms of geographical distance, but are large enough to sustain a range of services like schools and tertiary health care. Other communities might be closer to a city, but are so small that residents have to travel to access major services.

The second, and most recent, definition is the Accessibility/Remoteness Index for Australia (ARIA) (Department of Health and Aged Care 1999). The ARIA system is an accessibility index, based on how easy it is for people to reach certain services that are considered essential, but taken for granted by people living in more populated areas. Unlike the RRMAC, the ARIA uses a geographical approach to determine remoteness, so factors such as the socioeconomic status of populations or population size factors are not assessed (Department of Health and Aged Care 1999). The ARIA classification defines a set of 201 service centres, divided into five categories, distributed around Australia. Remoteness is interpreted as accessibility by road distance from a service centre. A grade of 1 on the ARIA classification means that the community is highly accessible, with relatively unrestricted access to a large range of goods and services and opportunities for interaction. At the other end, a grade of 5 means 'very remote', where there is a restricted ability to access (Department of Health and Aged Care 1999).

Regardless, the Brown family, who live 400km from the nearest major centre and only have access to a limited health service and small 10-bed hospital in their local town, are disadvantaged. In terms of isolation, distance, and accessibility to services, their situation and thus experiences of chronic and mental illness are very different to those who live in the city.

# The incidence of chronic illnesses in rural areas

Exactly how do the factors typical of rural life affect the experience of illness for Louise and her family? Firstly, there are significant health-related consequences of living outside a metropolitan area. Death rates in Australia rise with increasing remoteness, although this is largely explained by the higher proportions of Indigenous people living in remoter parts of Australia (Australian Institute of Health and Welfare 2003). Mortality rates from heart, stroke and vascular disease are slightly higher in remote areas than metropolitan areas (Australian Institute of Health and Welfare 2003). However, reports relating to cancer mortality between rural, remote and metropolitan areas are conflicting. Indigenous people are less likely to die of cancer than non-Indigenous rural Australians (Australian Institute of Health and Welfare 2000), probably because the health and psychosocial outcomes of Indigenous Australians are so poor that they do not reach an age where they are likely to develop cancer (Australian Institute of Health and Welfare 2000).

Like mortality rates in rural areas, morbidity levels also rise with increasing remoteness from major centres. Relatively poor access to health services, lower socioeconomic status and employment levels, harsher environments and higher occupational hazards explain many of these inequities (Australian Institute of Health and Welfare 2000). In addition, a number of personal risk factors, including higher alcohol consumption, smoking, and lack of exercise, are more prevalent in non-metropolitan areas (Australian Institute of Health and Welfare 2000).

One challenge that is especially confronting for people in rural and remote communities is that of privacy. Health problems which are 'unattractive'; for example, mental illness, and drug and alcohol problems, may be of particular concern in small communities since maintaining privacy can be almost impossible. Louise says that news of her cancer diagnosis travelled fast, and when she first came home after her surgery, she felt really self-conscious, because she thought everyone was looking at her, trying to work out which breast was 'real' and which was 'the falsie'.

As Louise makes clear, having to travel longer distances for specialist and primary health services is common for rural people in Australia. The time involved in travelling, the costs of travelling, being away from home and family/work responsibilities and accommodation costs impose significant economic and personal costs for rural Australians already burdened by the significant health problems discussed above (Eyles & Smith 1995, Hegney et al 2002, McCarthy et al 2002). In addition, relatively few rural people these days can afford the extra cost of health insurance, and for some, even the cost of fuel for transport to health services can be prohibitive (McCarthy & Hegney 1999). Consequently, even when rural women are faced with breast cancer, they may be reluctant to choose treatment options that involve expensive, prolonged and recurrent trips to a specialist health service.

For example, like Louise, less rural women (34%) in Australia in 1993 had breast-conserving treatment (lumpectomy) as compared to 42% of metropolitan women. Lumpectomy usually requires follow-up radiotherapy treatment, and these figures may reflect the inability or unwillingness of rural women who would prefer lumpectomies to access postoperative radiotherapy (Craft et al 1997). Since radiotherapy services are not generally available in rural areas, rural women who have lumpectomies to treat their breast cancer may need to travel to a tertiary health service, and be away from home for a number of weeks for their radiotherapy treatment (COSA

2001, Hegney et al 2002). Therefore rural women opt for more radical surgery, with serious long-term side effects such as lymphoedema and altered body image, over breast conserving surgery followed by radiotherapy. This preference is also influenced by the enormous financial burden and social upheaval necessitated by prolonged radiotherapy treatment.

# Issues regarding current models of rural health service delivery

Like Louise, many people with chronic illnesses in rural areas have comparatively restricted access to health services that would make their long-term illness experience more manageable. In recognition of this, in 2001, health professionals and consumers from regional and rural Australia gathered in Canberra to consider strategies to address the problem of inadequate services in rural areas for people with cancer. A number of key health service delivery issues that contribute to poorer long-term cancer outcomes were identified at the conference. These included (COSA 2001):

- *transport*, including problems with existing travel subsidy schemes which offer some financial compensation to help rural people meet the costs of travel for health care;

- *client support*, with a need to implement the breast cancer nurse and cancer nurse models nationally to ensure cancer survivors receive holistic and comprehensive care;

- *education and training*, with an identified need for more training for rural and remote area health professionals in the area of cancer diagnosis, treatment, and rehabilitation, so that residents of rural Australia can receive high quality care from their local health care professionals;

- *workforce planning*, with a need to attract and retain cancer specialists (medical, nursing and allied health) to rural areas which will mean more specialised care is available in rural areas;

- *networks*, with an identified problem being the lack of co-ordinated interaction between the large health services where many rural clients are treated initially, and the local health professionals who deliver their long-term care;

- *epidemiology*, particularly the need to examine cancer survival rates and outcomes in rural Australia;

- *access to services*, especially psychosocial support and the resulting differences in reported quality of life in rural and remote versus urban Australians;

- *reimbursement*, with a need for Medicare item numbers to be attached to specific rural services requiring significant travel and video-conference support; and

- *issues of national priority*, including the need to make specific cancer drugs available on the pharmaceutical benefits scheme, and the need to action radiation oncology proposals.

## Nursing in rural areas

It is worthwhile to briefly consider the role of nurses who work in rural areas, and the subsequent impact of rural nursing practice on the psychosocial aspects of caring for the chronically ill person. This is because rural nurses provide the bulk of health care outside of metropolitan areas, and some of you may choose to practise in these areas and care for rural people like the Brown family.

Depending on the context in which they practice, such as in a bush nursing post, in a small local hospital such as the one available to the Brown family, in a larger regional centre, or in community health, rural nurses can have a very different scope of practice from their metropolitan colleagues. A rural nurse is likely to be the first health professional immediately accessible to the Brown family because the town only has a visiting medical service. This is an enormous responsibility, as rural nurses are also expected to provide a wide variety of expert health services to other members of their community. Unfortunately, it is well recognised that rural nurses, no matter how willing they may be to provide this breadth of service, are often not educationally prepared to deliver the expert holistic care expected of them (McCarthy et al 2002). This occurs for a variety of reasons, mainly the lack of access to appropriate nursing education and issues of professional and geographical isolation (Hegney et al 1997). Furthermore, rural nurses tend, in the absence of formal education, to learn on the job or teach themselves the skills they need (McCarthy & Hegney 1999). People like Louise and Des, therefore, may not receive the level of psychosocial care they require.

However, many rural nurses spend their entire working lives in the one community, and are therefore positioned to deliver the type of 'womb to tomb' care that facilitates continuity of care and a truly holistic perspective (Hegney et al 1997). Given appropriate education and training, these nurses, with their enormous insight into the psychosocial and physical needs of the client and their family, are able to greatly enhance client outcomes. Many talk about the privilege of personally knowing their clients and their family intimately; their ability to adapt their practice to their clients' well-known psychosocial needs; and the professional satisfaction they gain by following up the long-term outcomes of nursing care (Hegney et al 1997). It is also evident from Louise's story that their clients greatly appreciate the quality of psychosocial care these nurses are able to give.

## Characteristics of rural people, rural life and the relationship with chronic illness outcomes

The media commonly report increasing poverty in rural areas, focusing on issues such as unemployment, decreasing farm incomes, drought, population drift, the closure of businesses and services, and the loss of farms by families who had always lived off the land (Coakes & Kelly 1997).

In Louise's case, she needed to stay close to home and work in her new job to contribute to the family income. Rural people with chronic illnesses often express this need. This means that even if a necessary health service is available, a lack of funds to access it may hinder their willingness to utilise it. Poverty is obviously an issue here, so you may wish to refer to Chapter 3, Class, Poverty and Illness: Intersecting Links, for a fuller consideration of the relationship between ill health and poverty.

Furthermore, many rural people define their health in terms of their ability to work, regardless of the presence of illness. This rural measure-ment of self-worth in terms of productivity also has implications for their psychosocial wellbeing when dealing with chronic illness (Viens 1997, Elliot-Schmidt & Strong 1997). Reluctance to consult health professionals may have a detrimental effect on their health outcomes. Many country people delay screening or treatment until it is financially viable for them to do so (McCarthy & Hegney 1999). In the case of cancer survivors who need regular life-long follow-up, this can have devastating consequences.

Despite the problems characteristic of rural areas, Louise's story also illustrates the benefits of country life. Rural life is not necessarily more difficult than urban living, nor is it necessarily a cause of ill health. For example, while Rogers-Clark (2002) found that the long-term survivors of breast cancer in her study faced particular difficulties relating to their rurality, such as geographical isolation, participants felt that the difficulties associated with being seriously ill in a rural setting were outweighed by the advantages of rural living. These included having access to highly effective informal support networks, and the sense of tranquillity available to them as rural dwellers. In fact, heath benefits can be substantial—such as access to clean air and a sense of space, as well as a sense of belonging and connection.

Similarly, in a study involving 394 participants in Queensland, Australia, women who lived in major rural towns reported fewer symptoms of stress, anxiety and depression than women in urban, remote and smaller rural areas (Rogers-Clark et al 1998). While women in smaller rural towns and remote areas reported more symptoms of psychological distress than women in major rural towns, the extent of their symptoms was similar to women in urban areas. This suggests that location by itself may not be an important factor in predicting the degree of emotional distress in a community (Rogers-Clark et al 1998). In a similar vein, another study found that rural women described themselves as healthier than urban women in Australia, despite having less access to health services and living in more hazardous environments (Wainer 1998).

Perhaps rural people have coping mechanisms that are not developed in people in the city. Louise certainly drew upon a number of strengths to empower her response to the psychological and social stressors of her chronic illness. These psychosocial strengths include a pride in the achievements and traditions of rural living, a culture of self-reliance, strong family connections, and a strong sense of community (Bigbee 1987, Hegney et al 2002). These are discussed in greater detail in the next section.

# Rural women's experiences of illness

Louise's narrative demonstrates that along with the trauma that any woman experiences when diagnosed with breast cancer, rural women may experience particular concerns because of their geographical location and, in particular, their distance from metropolitan areas and specialist health services. However, research that specifically examines rural women's experiences of cancer is extremely limited despite the abundance of literature about breast cancer and its effects on women.

One study in Queensland, Australia, though small and limited in scope, has shed some light on the particular concerns of rural women with breast cancer (McGrath et al 1999a, McGrath et al 1999b). Twenty-eight women participated in the study, using a structured telephone interview schedule. The participants' major concerns were similar to previous research outlining the concerns of women with breast cancer—fear of recurrence, physical concerns, and concerns about their family (McGrath et al 1999b). They were also asked questions relating to psychosocial support issues, including details relating to personal support, available and desired support, support from health professionals, and emotional, informational and practical support. The women in this study found that their distance from metropolitan areas led to hardships such as being separated from family and friends at a time of heightened vulnerability, having to travel long distances for follow-up care, and additional financial burdens arising from travel and accommodation costs. These combined hardships put pressure on marital and other family relationships. On a positive note, the women found significant support from within the informal support networks operating in rural areas. These networks included family, friends and community, and offered significant practical and emotional support to the women and their loved ones through the ordeal of breast cancer (McGrath et al 1999a).

Perhaps because of the absence of formal health support networks, rural women have developed a culture of self-reliance, independence and support from informal sources such as family, friends and the local community. This may affect their cancer experience in both positive and negative ways (Burman & Weinert 1997). For example, due to their reported self-reliance, rural women may be more reluctant to accept help from health professionals, despite having similar needs to urban women (Silveira & Winstead-Fry 1997, Bushy 1990). Similarly, stoicism and conservative gender attitudes are also well known social attributes in rural areas and may prevent rural women's use of health services (McCarthy & Hegney 1999). This more rigid definition of women's roles means that they may consider themselves more as service providers than service users, socialised to place the needs of others before their own. Therefore, when times are difficult on the land, and there is a chance that they can deal with the problem on their own, rural women may not prioritise their own health and may be reluctant to access the health services they need (Coakes & Kelly 1997). This propensity to meet role responsibilities before attending to one's own needs is not unique to rural women. However, rural women with multiple roles within their families and communities, as well as on their properties if they are farming women, may find it difficult to put aside these responsibilities even when their health is at risk. Like women everywhere, they are likely to place a strong emphasis on being with loved ones. For example, in one study, rural women with cancer feared separation from loved ones more than rural men with cancer (Burman & Weinert 1997).

Concerns about privacy and confidentiality may also be barriers to accessing help when rural women with breast cancer are having difficulties managing their illness and its consequences. Norms of self-reliance among rural people may mean that rural women feel as if they have failed if they seek assistance (Coakes & Kelly 1997). Furthermore, if a woman's emotional or physical trauma is related to family or relationship difficulties, difficulties with coping, self and body image problems, as well as her breast cancer, then concerns about confidentiality are likely to be critical. Professional commitments to confidentiality may have little meaning to the woman in a small and close-knit community, who must interact socially with health practitioners who have sensitive knowledge of the woman and her family.

On the positive side, it is evident from Louise's narrative that the informal yet highly effective systems of support available to rural people are valuable for rural people with chronic illnesses (Brown 1990, McGrath et al 1999a). Kate Brown (1990, p 52) wrote of the 'paradox' of rural health, whereby rural dwellers define health as the capacity to stay independent, yet believe that they are able to achieve good health, and therefore their independence by staying 'connected' to the community by being involved in community activities. Hence, individuals in a rural community contribute to their own health by staying connected, and it is this very strategy that also ensures the health of the community. This 'connected independence' is apparent in the stories of participants in Rogers-Clark's study (2002).

This 'connected independence' came to be most important for the entire Brown family, who found, to their distress, that Louise's cancer was not to be the only health-related adversity they were to face. Des, the youngest son of the family, began to confront the difficulties associated with mental illness.

# The issues of mental illnesses in rural areas

## Case study—Des's story

Des loved the farm, and envisaged spending his whole life working on it, as his parents and grandparents had done before him. However, the drought had been devastating. It had brought about a rural recession as a result of a decline in the agricultural economy. Whilst the family had been able to manage for several years, it had come to a point where the bank was considering foreclosing on the farm. Despite every attempt to avoid this, the inevitable occurred, and Des and his family lost the farm which had been owned by his family for generations.

Des and his parents moved into the small local town as they did not want to leave the area. Des saw himself as a 'bushy'; it was all he knew. As the surrounding farms continued to downsize or foreclose in the area, the unemployment rate increased in the town. Des could not find a job, despite the fact that he was willing to do any work. He began to lose hope. Louise and Bob noticed that Des was different to his normal self. He was becoming aggressive and getting involved in fights, especially after spending a few hours at the pub, an increasingly common pastime for him. He didn't want to talk to anyone and gradually became more and more withdrawn. Two days after he told Louise that 'nothing mattered anymore' he was admitted to the local hospital and diagnosed with severe clinical depression, but only after Louise had been up to the hospital and expressed her fear that he was about to commit suicide. Unfortunately, getting Des to go into hospital was quite a challenge, and in the end the police had to be called in to help. Des was then sent to an acute psychiatric unit, three hours drive away, for specialist treatment.

In a twelve-month period, almost one in five Australians will experience a mental health problem (McLennan 1998). Rural people are particularly at risk for poor mental health (AHMC 1999), with rural and remote communities targeted by the Commonwealth Department of Health and Aged Care as a priority group in need of high quality mental health services (DHAC 2000a). According to Wainer & Chesters (2000) particular mental health risk factors found in rural areas include the relative poverty due to economic conditions, negative life experiences and lack of control over work, and life in general. Alcohol and other drug abuse, lack of access to education and employment opportunities, changing gender roles, and sexuality issues may partly explain the higher rates of depression and suicide in rural and remote areas (Wainer & Chesters 2000).

The stigma of mental illness within small and often ill-informed groups, and the introspection of small communities, can negatively effect an individual's capacity to cope when they are unwell, and perhaps more so, if affected by mental health problems (Judd & Humphreys 2001). Des really did not understand what was happening to him in the time before his hospitalisation. His mother had suggested to him that maybe he was getting depressed, and needed help, but he refused to listen to 'that rubbish'. The combination of misperception about what constitutes mental health problems coupled with the tradition of stoicism and self-reliance may well increase the distress felt by some rural people when dealing with adversity.

Issues of confidentiality, raised earlier this chapter in relation to Louise, are also highly relevant for rural men. Buckley & Lower (2002) found, in their study of rural men's uptake of health services, that men who were not especially worried about privacy issues were 2.57 times more likely to access health services than men who had serious concerns about lack of confidentiality.

# Depression and suicide in rural men

One reality of rural living is an increased risk for suicide in men. According to Strong et al (1998), suicide is one of the major causes of injury-related death in Australian males, with much higher rates compared to females. Men are more likely to attempt suicide by hanging, carbon monoxide poisoning and firearms, which are more likely to be successful than, for example, taking an overdose of medication.

Reasons why rural men commit suicide cannot easily be explained, because suicidal behaviour is not simply a response to single stress but related and compounding vulnerabilities (DHAC 2000b). In relation to rural men, it is apparent that the increase in stressors relating to their current situation, such as drought and economic downturn, can expand into wider problems, such as family distress and personal losses. From Des's story, we can surmise that the loss of the family farm meant for him the loss of the future he had planned, which was clearly devastating.

Depression has been defined as the most common mental illness associated with suicide (Beautrais 1998 cited in DHAC 2000b). Depression can result in a reduction in the capacity of individuals to cope in difficult times and to seek out the treatment that is required. We see evidence of this in Des's story. His grief at losing the family farm, and then being unable to find employment, was doubtless a major reason for his depression. However, his capacity to deal with these difficulties was reduced by his ensuing depression, and his only way of responding was to start to consume a lot of alcohol.

Unresolved or untreated depression compounds, and is often the pre-cursor to a range of somatic illnesses and disintegration within the domestic environment. Des became withdrawn at home, and hence his family relation-ships suffered. Louise and Bob were extremely worried about Des, but they found his behaviour at home became very difficult to live with, especially when he was drunk. Bob was worried about the effect this was having on Louise. He knew she still worried that her breast cancer might recur, and losing the farm had really distressed her. Now Des's problems were again putting the entire family under a lot of pressure.

With advances in treatment of mental illnesses, happily many conditions can be successfully treated or managed. This management, which not only promotes better mental health outcomes for individuals, can also have a positive effect on their immediate family (Judd et al 2001). Louise and Bob had felt relieved when Des had been admitted to hospital, because they could relax knowing he was in good hands. They could see that Des's depression was lifting with the treatment he was receiving in hospital.

After a month, Des returned home in much better spirits, and with renewed hope. His parents noted that he had started a daily practice of writing in a diary, and also practising meditation. In discussions with his parents, he revealed that he was thinking about applying to study nursing, after a number of discussions with a couple of the nurses at the mental health unit. He'd always liked people, and he thought that living through his mother's cancer, and his own depression, had given him insights which would really be helpful in nursing. He had found out that there was a significant shortage of mental health nurses in the bush, so hoped that after his studies were finished he'd be able to return to his own community to live and work.

Des's experiences of recovering from his depression were echoed in the findings of a research project exploring resilience in rural men at risk of suicide (Hegney et al 2003). Ten rural men who had been through difficult times and may have considered suicide at some point in their lives participated in this study, which found that there were a number of factors which partici-pants considered to be helpful in getting through tough times. Personal factors included positive thinking, taking control, being self-aware, appreciating what they had and hoping that things would get better, and seeking meaning through a sense of purpose and/or religious beliefs. Having support, such as access to information, professional support and treatment, having someone to talk to, and relying on family and friends were also seen as very helpful. Being needed by others was a boost. Finally, participants noted that making some sort of life change, or getting away for a while, was really important.

The results of this study, and the stories of the men participating in it, have been widely sought by individuals and groups seeking to support rural men through difficult times. This was because of the positive nature of the study, which focused on men's resilience in managing their depression rather than focusing only on the problems they were experiencing. Resilience is a growing area of interest for nurses, and is explored in more depth in Chapter 11, Journeys Through Illness: Suffering and Resilience. Readers should also refer to Chapter 4, Gender and Illness, for further discussion of men's health issues.

## Conclusion

Most discussions of about rural and remote health identify only the difficulties associated with rural living. This is understandable, given the well-documented problems in rural communities, which include the downturn in rural economies, a decreasing population, and lack of services (Australian Institute of Health and Welfare 2000, Humphreys & Rolley 1991). It is ironic that, in the recent drive to highlight the significant social and economic problems that rural communities are experiencing, the positive aspects of rural living are dismissed and replaced with images of decline and hardship. Inadvertently, this could actually be adding to the declining populations of rural areas, and the inability of rural communities to attract professionals like nurses to their areas. In relation to rural people living with illness, it is vital that any interventions seek to build on the strengths of rural communities in relation to lifestyle and support, rather than assuming that rural communities are defined by the absence of specialised services.

## Tutorial questions

1. Given the strengths of Australian rural women identified in this chapter, can you think of practical ways you could build on these to help them manage their chronic illnesses?

2. The many factors that contribute to the inappropriate management of one chronic disease (breast cancer) in rural areas have been identified in this chapter. Identify another chronic disease common to men in rural areas; brainstorm the contributing factors to this condition; and provide two practical solutions for each factor that might assist rural men to overcome them.

3. This chapter has considered depression as an example of a mental illness common amongst men in rural areas. Can you think of other mental health issues which may create difficulties for rural people?

4.  Have you considered a career in rural nursing? Identify the factors which would encourage you to work in a rural area as well as the factors which would discourage you.

# References

Australian Health Ministers' Conference 1999 *Healthy Horizons: a Framework for Improving the Health of Rural, Regional and Remote Australians, 1999–2003.* Commonwealth Department of Health and Aged Care, Canberra

Australian Institute of Health and Welfare (AIHW) 2003 *Rural, Regional and Remote Health: A Study on Mortality, Summary of Findings, Mortality Series No 3.* CanPrint, Canberra

—2000 *Australia's Health 2000.* Canberra: Australian Institute of Health and Welfare

Bigbee JL 1987 Stressful life events among women: A rural-urban comparison. The *Journal of Rural Health* 3(1):39–51

Brown K 1990 Connected Independence: A paradox of rural health? *Journal of Rural Community Psychology* 11(1):51–63

Buckley D, Lower T 2002 Factors influencing the utilisation of health services by rural men. *Australian Health Review* 25(2):11–15

Burman ME, Weinert C 1997 Rural dwellers' cancer fears and perceptions of cancer treatment. *Public Health Nursing* 14(5):272–279

Bushy A 1990 Rural US Women: Traditions and transitions affecting health care. *Health Care for Women International.* 11:503–513

Clinical Oncology Society of Australia (COSA) 2001 *Cancer in the Bush: Optimising Clinical Services.* Report and recommendations from a meeting held at the National Convention Centre, Canberra, 8th and 9th of March

Coakes SJ and Kelly GJ 1997 Community competence and empowerment: Strategies for rural change in women's health service planning and delivery. *Australian Journal of Rural Health* 5:26–30

Commonwealth Department of Health and Aged Care 2000(a) *National Action Plan for Promotion, Prevention and Early Intervention for Mental Health 2000.* Commonwealth of Australia, Canberra

Commonwealth Department of Health and Aged Care 2000(b) *LIFE: Living is for everyone. A framework for prevention of suicide and self-harm in Australia.* Commonwealth of Australia, Canberra

Craft PS, Primrose JG, Lindner JA, McManus PR 1997 Surgical management of breast cancer in Australian women in 1993: analysis of Medicare statistics. *Medical Journal of Australia* 166,(June), pp 626–629

Department of Health and Aged Care 1999 *Accessibility/Remoteness Index of Australia.* AGPS, Canberra

Department of Primary Industries and Energy 1991 *Rural, Remote and Metropolitan Areas Classification: 1991 Census Edition.* Department of Primary Industries and Energy, Canberra

Elliot-Schmidt R and Strong J 1997 The concept of wellbeing in a rural setting: understanding health and illness. *Australian Journal of Rural Health* 5(2):59–63

Eyles R and Smith B 1995 Rural health in Queensland: a changing focus. *Australian Journal of Rural Health* 3:18–22

Hegney D, McCarthy A, Martin-McDonald K, Pearce S, Rogers-Clark C 2002 *An Analysis of the Needs of People with Cancer Travelling from Toowoomba and South*

*West Queensland to Brisbane for Radiotherapy Treatment.* Centre for Rural and
Remote Area Health, USQ, Toowoomba

Hegney D, Pearson A, McCarthy A 1997 *The Role and Function of the Rural Nurse.*
Royal College of Nursing Australia, Canberra

Hegney D, Gorman, McCullagh, Pearce, Rogers-Clark, Weir 2003 *Rural men getting
through adversity: Stories of resilience.* Centre for Rural and Remote Area Health
and Welfare, Canberra

Humphreys J and Rolley F 1991 *Health and Health Care in Rural Australia.* University
of New England, Armidale

Judd F, Humphreys J 2001 Mental health issues for rural and remote Australians.
*Australian Journal of Rural Health* 9(5):254–258

Judd F, Jackson H, David J, Cockram A, Kimiti A, Allen N, Murray G, Kyrios M,
Hodgins G 2001, Improving access for rural Australians to treatment for anxiety
and depression: The University of Melbourne Depression and Anxiety Research
and Treatment Group—Bendigo Health Care Group Initiative, *Australian Journal
of Rural Health,* 9:91–96

McCarthy A, Hegney D 1999 Rural and Remote Palliative Care. In Aranda S and
O'Connor M (eds) *Palliative Care Nursing: a Guide to Practic*e. Ausmed
Publications, Melbourne

McCarthy A, Brodribb TR, Brown L, Gilbar P, Hegney D, Raith L, Swales J 2002 *The
Chemotherapy Education Needs of Nurses Working in Rural and Remote Areas of
Queensland.* Centre for Rural and Remote Area Health, USQ, Toowoomba

McGrath P, Patterson C, Yates P, Trealoar S, Oldenburg B and Loos C 1999a A study
of postdiagnosis breast cancer concerns for women living in rural and remote
Queensland. Part II: Support Issues. *Australian Journal of Rural Health* 7:43–52

McGrath P, Patterson C, Yates P, Trealoar S, Oldenburg B and Loos C 1999b A study
of postdiagnostic breast cancer concerns for women living in rural and remote
Queensland. Part 1: Personal Concerns. *Australian Journal of Rural Health* 7:34–42

McLennan A 1998 *Mental Health and Wellbeing: Profile of Adults, Australia 1997.*
Australian Bureau of Statistics, Canberra

O'Connor-Flemming M and Parker D 2001 *Health Promotion: Principles and Practice in
the Australian Context,* 2nd edn. Allen & Unwin, St Leonards NSW

Reid M, Solomon S 1992 *Improving Australia's Rural Health and Aged Care Services.*
AGPS, Canberra

Rogers-Clark C, Bramston P and Hegney D 1998 Women's emotional health and
wellbeing: an urban/rural comparison, in 4th Biennial Australian Rural and
Remote Health Scientific Conference Proceedings, ed Hegney D, Toowomba,
Queensland, Australia

Rogers-Clark, C 2002 Resilient Survivors: Rural Women Who Have Lived Through
Breast Cancer, Doctoral Dissertation. University of Southern Queensland, Australia

Silveira JM, Winstead-Fry P 1997 The needs of patients with cancer and their
caregivers in rural areas. *Oncological Nursing Forum* 24(1):71–76

Strong K, Trickett P, Titulaer I, Bhatia K 1998 *Health in rural and remote Australia.* The
first report of the Australian Institute of Health and Welfare on Rural Health.
Australian Institute of Health and Welfare, Canberra

Viens C 1997 Developing expertise in the rural environment. *Canadian Nurse* 93(2):39–42

Wainer J 1998 Rural Women's Health. *Australian Journal of Primary Health Interchange*
4(3):80–88

Wainer J, Chesters J 2000 'Rural mental health: neither romanticism nor despair',
*Australian Journal of Rural Health* 8:141–147

# Chapter 8

## Constructions of Chronic Illness

*Sally Wellard and Lenore Beddoes*

**This chapter:**

- the factors that influence the current biomedical and psychosocial approach to chronic illness;
- existing knowledge about the trajectory of chronic illnesses, quality of life and compliance;
- critically examines the effect of the concepts of science and individualism on and the response of health care organisations to chronic illness;
- explains the role of normalisation and stigma in chronic illness;
- explores the characteristics of the experience of stigma; and
- identifies challenges for nurses in developing relevant practices for chronic illness care.

Chronic illness has become increasingly common in developed countries with the decline in mortality rates from acute and infectious illness. This decline is associated with improved sanitation, vaccination (Gerhardt 1990, Hinman 1998) and public health surveillance (Callaghan & Berg 2002, Strauss 1984). In recent times, chronic illness has been referred to as an epidemic accounting for 80% of the burden of disease in Australia (AIHW 2002). It therefore contributes to high social and economic costs for both the community and individuals. It is important that nurses develop a deep understanding of the psychosocial experiences associated with chronic illness, which will assist them to provide sensitive and appropriate nursing care aimed at helping people to 'live well' with their chronic illness.

This chapter considers peoples' experiences of chronic illness by considering the sociocultural factors influencing perceptions of, and responses to, those with chronic illness. Hence, this chapter provides a broad discussion about chronic illness that is complemented by further discussion of specific aspects of the illness experience in Chapter 9, Psychosocial Aspects of Pain and Fatigue, Chapter 10, Living with Loss and Grief, and Chapter 11, Journeys Through Illness: Suffering and Resilience.

A key feature of this chapter is discussion of the impact of 'science', 'individualism' and 'normalisation' on the experience of chronic illness. The systems of care currently available for those with chronic illness are also discussed. A focus of the chapter will be the identification of people with chronic illness as 'abnormal', with a subsequent experience of stigma that deepens and extends the difficulties of managing illness as a part of life. Using a case study, aspects of stigma in the context of chronic illness will be explored.

Previous studies have focused on the sufferer of chronic illness. There is a need now to consider the wider social context to better understand chronic illness, which can be done through an examination of prevalent discourses. The work of French philosopher Michel Foucault (1972, 1975a, b) has been useful in exploring 'discourses' that are central to our current views of chronic illness. A discourse is a way of thinking, speaking or writing about something or things which has shared meaning to those using that system. Some of these systems are entrenched within societies, and influence how we view the world. They influence the language we use about chronic illness and the practices we develop to manage those illnesses. For example, a 'medical discourse' encourages us to think about illness from a biophysical perspective, and to target the defective cells, tissues or organs that have caused the illness. Nursing discourses, on the other hand, ask us to not only consider the physiological management of the disease, but to also consider the person with the illness from a holistic perspective.

Our ways of knowing and being in the world are not simply governed by one discourse, but rather many competing ones. This is the case with our ways of thinking about and responding to chronic illness, where a review of the research and literature about chronic illnesses reveals three main groups of discourses. These are the discourses of individualism (with a focus on the individual), science (with a focus on searching for truth through objective reasoned thought), and normalisation (with a focus on the average as normal or 'right'). These dominant discourses in turn influence the practices of nurses and all other health practitioners.

# Case study

Three years ago when Joanne was 26, she became concerned when she started to experience signs of Type 1 diabetes mellitus (thirst, excessive urination). Joanne's general practitioner (GP) established her diagnosis and, together with a practice nurse, assisted Joanne to become independent in her management of blood glucose monitoring and insulin injections. Joanne, although appearing to cope with the practical aspects of management of her blood glucose level, did have some difficulty adjusting to the changes that had occurred since her diagnosis was made.

Joanne was relieved when she was first diagnosed; she finally knew the reason why she had been feeling so ill. At the same time, she worried about what this might mean for her career as a police officer. Joanne found her job to be stressful at times because of the long hours, responsibility and the physical activity involved. She wondered how her superior officer and colleagues would react when, and if, she informed them. She decided to hide her diagnosis, but was seen by a colleague when giving herself a dose of insulin. It was embarrassing and there were initially some accusations that she was taking illicit drugs.

She considered how diabetes might affect her social and recreational pastimes. Joanne enjoyed rock climbing and would often spend weekends away with a group of her friends and her boyfriend, Andy. She also thought about diabetes and its impact on her relationship, sexual activity, and her decision to have children or not—if the time were right, would she be able to have a 'normal' pregnancy and would diabetes affect her baby?

Joanne had regular follow-up visits and felt able to discuss these issues with her health care team. She also became aware of some very helpful support groups and websites available on the Internet, which provide people with Type 1 diabetes with the opportunity to connect on-line. She felt relieved to know that there were people who were grappling with similar issues and who needed answers to the same questions.

Following initial stabilisation, Joanne's blood glucose levels have remained elevated for the past several months, despite her adherence to the treatment regimen. Ongoing visits to her health team have resulted in constant revision of her insulin program and Joanne recently had her insulin regimen reviewed by a consultant endocrinologist. In Joanne's words, 'When I visited the endocrinologist it felt a bit like I had to prove that I'd been monitoring my blood sugar, eating the right diet and giving myself the correct insulin doses. It turns out that I might have developed a resistance to the insulin that I take. To tell you the truth, I have wondered if the insulin has been working at all for a while now, and I nearly stopped taking it. I've altered my diet, been aware of my activity levels and regularly administered the insulin and my blood sugar levels are still not normal.'

Joanne has been trying to come to terms with the limited efficacy of her treatment and is interested in exploring new treatment options with her endocrinologist and GP. She related that once the team realised that she really wanted to get her blood sugars under control, and that she was trying desperately to manage this, the level of their support seemed to change. They seemed more willing to try every avenue to assist her.

# Approaches to understanding chronic illnesses

The literature discussing chronic illness deals with a variety of pathophysiology and psychosocial perspectives. In this section, a brief note is made of the pathophysical perspectives on chronic illness, leading on to a consideration of the manifestations of chronic illness, quality of life and compliance issues.

## Pathophysiology in focus

Medical literature relating to chronic illnesses, such as diabetes, is largely focused on the investigation of the pathophysiology of specific diseases, and treatment options. The primary aim of treatment is to reverse, if possible, the course of illness and restore the patient to a normal state of health, thereby affecting a 'cure'. Where cure is not attainable, treatment becomes focused on minimising the impact of the disease. This is usually achieved through 'symptom control'. This focus inevitably leads to a view of the person with disease as a physiological entity. In Joanne's case, for example, the use of insulin as a treatment is focused on supplying this hormone to enable glucose to be transported from the blood into body cells where it can be used for cellular processes.

The medical approach toward the exploration of any disease is the scientific method, using 'normal' populations as controls. Controls in this way are used as a contrast to the disease state, differentiating people with the disease state from 'normal' individuals. Medical research, with a focus on 'curing' disease states, does not usually attend to the whole person with a chronic illness for whom a cure is not possible. This can mean that the 'care and dependency needs' of those with chronic illness are ignored (Cooper 1990). Simply, people with chronic illnesses are seen as the illness, rather than a person with an illness.

## Psychosocial views

Psychosocial approaches to chronic illness have sought to analyse the social and psychological manifestations of chronic illness. Four major themes identified within the psychosocial area of inquiry are:

- manifestations of chronic illness;
- the 'mapping' of illness trajectories;
- the evaluation of quality of life; and
- the exploration of the notion of compliance.

### Manifestations of chronic illness

Strauss et al (1984) characterised chronic illness as an experience of multiple problems that may change but do not go away. Chronic illness is marked by periodic medical crises. Preventing and controlling these crises requires the person with the illness to engage in planning as well as developing complex social arrangements to manage the upheaval involved. When Joanne in our case study first developed Type 1 diabetes mellitus, she experienced symptoms caused by hyperglycaemia, such as polydipsia (thirst), polyphagia (hunger) and polyuria (increased urination). Through these symptoms Joanne experienced a type of medical crisis that had a tremendous impact on her life.

Chronic illness creates a demand to manage treatment regimens. A major endeavour for chronically ill persons is to manage the symptoms of their illness. Adhering to the treatment plan was identified by Strauss et al (1984) as a major means of attaining this. Sometimes, however, this is not enough. In addition to their medical regimens, ill people will often seek to supplement their regimens with alternative treatments if they discover that their symptoms are persisting.

In order to manage, people with chronic illness reorder time to juggle the management of both their illness and their lives. This is part of trying to maintain a 'normal life'. A key strategy in living with chronic illness, according to Strauss et al (1984), is normalisation. People hide and conceal their disease from others, trying to pass themselves as 'normal', an idealised notion of being the same as the rest of the presumably 'normal' population. For instance, Joanne attempted to hide and conceal her Type 1 diabetes mellitus from her colleagues, wanting to appear the same as her peers.

## Mapping of trajectories

The second major area of psychosocial investigation has been the idea of 'illness trajectory' as a way of understanding the complex path of chronic illness (Glaser & Strauss 1967). A trajectory is a pathway, and the notion of progress along that pathway is implicit in the term. Trajectories have been explored from the perspective of those involved (the ill and their carers) and assist in predicting the rate of symptom progression, the types of crises that may occur, and the patterns and variability in specific disease development. The complexity of some illnesses, together with an increase in technological treatments, means that there are very many more possible trajectories (Lubkin 1998).

Mapping trajectories has been of interest to many with Rolland (1987) developing the early work about adaptation in chronic illness. He described four basic classifications that are very helpful in identifying key features of the psychosocial aspects of chronic disease: 'onset', the rate at which the disease occurs; 'course' of the disease categorised as either progressive, constant or relapsing/episodic; 'outcome' of the disease on life span; and the 'degree of incapacitation'. The onset of Joanne's diabetes was gradual, with symptoms slowly becoming more noticeable. The course of her disease has been episodic. After diagnosis, she had some months of stabilisation, but thereafter her blood sugar levels became quite erratic, causing significant concern. The degree of incapacitation experienced by Joanne has been significant enough to create stress for her, as she has attempted to juggle her work and personal lives with her new dietary, exercise and medication regime. However, she has managed to keep working and pursue an active recreational life, so in one sense the incapacity she has experienced thus far has been slight.

Along with these classifications, it is also helpful to think about the time phases within chronic illness trajectories. Rolland (1987) identified three such time phases. First, there is the 'crisis' phase, which is the period before and immediately surrounding diagnosis, where learning to live with symptoms and illness-related demands takes place. This was a difficult time for Joanne, who found that her diabetes had consequences for her work and private life. She experienced a lot of anxiety as she tried to accommodate her life around her newly diagnosed disease, and she worried about the long-term consequences. Second is the 'chronic' phase, the time span between initial diagnosis and the final time phase where the key task is to continue as normal a life as possible in the face of the abnormality of having a chronic illness where the outcomes are uncertain (Rolland 1987). Joanne wondered whether she would ever be able to have children, and was worried that her police work would suffer. Nevertheless, she made relevant lifestyle changes and monitored her blood sugar levels in an effort to manage her diabetes. Third, the 'terminal' phase is marked by issues surrounding grief and death. Not everyone with chronic illness will move into this phase, because some chronic illnesses, such as arthritis, are not life-threatening, whilst other diseases such as diabetes, if carefully managed, will not necessarily lead to death.

This model, and others like it, are useful but have some limitations. Perhaps the most significant problem is that such models can be used as an indicator of what is normal in adapting to chronic illness. Hence, where a person's response to chronic illness does not match the model, these responses may be seen as abnormal. Expectations also tend to accompany the classification approach. That is, individuals are expected to conform to predefined trajectories. Joanne, for example, with a diagnosis of Type 1 diabetes mellitus and her seemingly poor glycaemic control, was interpreted as non-compliant with treatment.

Moving away from a classificatory approach, Strauss and others (Corbin & Strauss 1991; Strauss et al 1984) argued that trajectories of illness are also strongly linked to the ill person's perceptions of events, as well as the physiological manifestations of their disease. Many diseases have fairly predictable trajectories, whilst other diseases are relatively uncertain. Whatever the trajectory, an ill person seeks to locate themselves within it. They are aware of the phases and changes in manifestations of their disease and are vigilant of symptom change as a means of tracking the course of their illness.

There are a growing number of publications from people with chronic illnesses who offer an alternative view of trajectories—discussing the journey of living with a chronic illness. Register (1987), for example, has a long-standing chronic illness, and described the journey from diagnosis through to finding new ways of living. This journey requires learning the politics of being an ill individual in a world of health-centred people. Initially, diagnosis of illness may be a time of elation, because finally the ill person feels that their concerns about the symptoms they have been experiencing have been legitimised. Diagnosis provides a tangible position from which the ill person can relate to the problems they are experiencing. It is noticeable, for example, that Joanne experienced feelings of 'relief' when she was initially diagnosed and had an explanation for why she had felt unwell.

From the elation of having a name for their problem, many people move through a process of grieving for the loss of their health and lifestyle. They frequently experience a preoccupation with self, focusing on the impact of the illness on all aspects of their life. As we've already noted, Joanne did just that. She considered many of her life ambitions in a new light, and wondered how having diabetes would affect her plans for the future as well as her present life.

After the initial diagnostic phase, chronically ill people experience stigma, which is frequently reinforced through association with others who are chronically ill. Being labelled by the disease they experience and the treatments they use, people with chronic illness are set apart from others. The 'etiquette' of chronic illness demands that chronically ill persons try to pass themselves as healthy or at least conform to societal expectations of the sick role. Social interaction with others constantly demands explanation of why the ill person is not the same as everyone else, why they look different, why they eat differently, why they walk or talk differently. The demand for explanation is a constant reminder of not being 'normal' (Register 1987). Ill people try to create as near a 'normal' appearance as possible to reduce the degree of stigma experienced.

## Assessing quality of life

Quality of life is seen as an important aspect of chronic illnesses. What quality of life actually means, however, is not clearly defined (Fries & Spitz 1990, Garratt et al 2002). Frequently, quality of life has been equated with the quality of the outcomes of various available treatments, and often physical, mental and social indicators as well as symptoms are assessed (Sanders et al 1998). Morbidity and mortality have been used to describe the quality of life outcomes but, as Burckhardt et al (1989) argued, the subjective perceptions of people with chronic illness need to be included if therapeutic nursing interventions are to enhance quality of life. In other words, it is not appropriate to measure quality of life, nor consider how nursing care can improve a person's quality of life, without actually asking that person to identify what is important for them in relation to their quality of life.

Interestingly, Molzahn and colleagues (1997) found that nurses rated quality of life lower than patients. This demonstrates a poor fit between consumer and health professional perceptions of needs in chronic illness management (Rasmussen, Wellard & Nankurvis 2001, Wellard & Rushton 2002, Wellard & Street 1999). It suggests that nurses may be focused on the problems associated with living with a chronic illness, but not with the resilience that people with chronic illness demonstrate in relation to managing their health problems. This is a topic that will be explored in more depth in Chapter 11, Journeys Through Illness: Suffering and Resilience.

## Compliance

Compliance with treatment has been the fourth major area of psychosocial inquiry relating to chronic illness. Health professionals view the successful management of chronic illness as reliant on patients' adherence to treatment regimens. Treatment regimens require patients to change the way in which they manage aspects of their life and can range from very simple to extremely complex routines.

The term 'compliance' infers patient submission to the medical (health professional) advice in relation to taking medication, following diets, or executing lifestyle changes (Vermeire et al 2001). Kyngäs (2000) refers to compliance as an active, intentional and responsible process of health care. It is estimated that compliance rates in chronic illness vary from 80% (Kyngäs et al 2000) to 50% (Cameron & Gregor 1987, Turk & Rudy 1991), depending on how compliance is defined and measured (Hailey & Moss 2000).

Non-compliance has been noted as having severe consequences, including exacerbation and progression of disability (Turk & Rudy 1991). A failure to follow treatment regimens can result in patients needing emergency treatments, and hospitalisation to re-establish a stable condition (Lamping & Campbell 1990). Consequently, medical non-compliance creates an additional economic burden on the health care system (Vermeire et al 2001). It has been argued that predicting the degree of compliance would allow clinicians to explore alternative strategies that would lead to increased patient compliance. Therefore, the surveillance of compliance has become an important feature of clinical practice.

Physiological and biochemical tests are frequently used to measure compliance (Fielding & Duff 1999). It is anticipated that if patients are compliant, then their test results will show the effects of following the treatment regimen. However, variations in these levels may not always indicate non-compliance. Changes in the illness state and variability in the treatment may contribute to fluctuations from the expected (Lamping & Campbell 1990). In the case of unstable diabetes, frequently attributed to poor compliance, Tanenberg (2001) reported that insulin resistance accounted for many reported cases of non-compliance in people with diabetes, as we see in Joanne's case. This means that she, and many other patients, may be erroneously labelled as non-complaint. Joanne felt she was judged as non-compliant before it was realised that her unstable blood sugar levels were due to insulin resistance. She said she felt that she received more supportive care once it was realised that she was adhering to the treatment regimen that had been ordered for her.

Current definitions of compliance infer a relationship of authority and power of one individual (medical and health professionals) over another (the patient) (Kontz 1989, Vermeire et al 2001). Compliance needs to be redefined to incorporate the patients' right to choose not to adopt treatment regimens. Nurses often speak of patient-centred care. However, efforts to encourage patients to be compliant suggest a paternalistic (father-like) approach (Fielding & Duff 1999, Kontz 1989, Vermiere et al 2001). It appears that the work of Kelly and May (1982), who identified the consequence of non-compliance by patients was to be labelled by health workers as 'bad patients', remains valid in current practice.

Nurses and patients may not think about compliance in the same ways. Patients evaluate and adopt treatments using social rather than health criteria, such as the financial costs associated with treatment, family expectations, the personal relationship they have with their doctor (Cameron & Gregor 1987) and a belief in the effectiveness of the treatment (Turk & Kerns 1985). Thorne (1990) identified two explanations patients give for non-compliance with treatments. First, patients may not trust the quality of decisions made by their health team, and so do not trust the treatment regimen given to them. Second, the need to maintain relationships with health care personnel prohibits total withdrawal. For example, Joanne could think that whilst she wants to continue her visits to the diabetic nurse at the hospital, she checks the recommendations she is given by conducting her own research on the Internet, and then makes her own decisions about what she will do. In this example, non-compliance serves as a strategy that allows the patient to exercise some control.

# Thinking about normal vs abnormal

Throughout the range of work relating to chronic illness, individualism and science predominate. The importance of these ways of seeing chronic illness experiences is evidenced in both the methods employed to investigate chronic illness and the findings arising from the use of those methods. The idea of normalisation is supported by and interwoven in both views of individualism and science.

## Individualism

Individualism refers to the valuing of individual interests over collective interests, where individual autonomy is argued as central. Individualism embraces notions of personal freedom, individual rights to self-determination and ownership, all of which have been very highly valued in western societies (Abercrombie, Hill & Turner 1986, O'Connor & Shimizu 2002, Tesh 1990). Accompanying the rights of individualism are obligations to demonstrate responsibility for individual actions. The freedom of self-determination becomes restrained by ideas of normal behaviour, where individuals are expected to conform to societal norms.

Within nursing and medical discourses, individualism predominates and can be seen in the focus of health care with individual patients. The 'patient', rather than the individual person or their family, become the object of nursing and medical interest. An interesting feature of this is that whilst the individual is seen as most important, each patient is always being compared with a population of individuals who have that specific complaint. For example, Joanne's nurse said to her at one stage that 'I expected your blood sugar levels to have settled by now. In my experience that's what happens with most patients.' In this way, the ideal 'individual' acts as a mechanism for control, as we examine and compare patients with the 'average' individual and reinforce expected norms.

One consequence of individualism is a shifting of 'blame' for being different to the average to the person who appears different (Lowenberg 1995). Individuals become 'responsible' for the cause of their illness because they are considered autonomous. Since Joanne's blood sugar levels were not stabilising, it was initially assumed by her nurse, general practitioner and endocrinologist that she was to blame. It took quite some time for an alternative explanation (insulin resistance) to be accepted. This is an example of what is known as 'victim blaming'.

Individualism has infiltrated many aspects of health care. Health promotion and education have become strategies for encouraging individual compliance to expected norms, and are used to show individuals the purported errors in their life choices that have led to ill health and to urge for change in those choices. This view does not acknowledge a social context in which health is experienced (Crawford 1984, Lowenberg 1995, Tesh 1990). Whilst individuals can seldom alter their social context, they are likely to accept this blame because they have learnt the societal values of individual responsibility.

## The promise of science

In Western society, there is a predominant belief that science will provide the truth or the answers to any problems posed about chronic illness. 'Medical miracles' are highlighted in the media, and specific television programs have been devised that discuss how medical innovations will improve illness outcomes. This faith in science has permeated most aspects of our social life, creating an effect of unquestioning acceptance of medical models that focus on the pathophysiologic aspects of illness whilst excluding the subjective experiences of the chronically ill.

## Living with Illness

The outcomes of medical research are used to underpin practice as well as influencing theoretical knowledge about chronic illness. Other ways of knowing about chronic illness, such as the wisdom of those living with a chronic illness, may be overlooked. This means that nurses who seek to enhance their knowledge about particular health problems are likely to find a wealth of information about the biomedical aspects of that problem, but a paucity of information about what it is like to live with the illness.

### Normalisation

Health care workers have promoted norms for patients 'in order to establish and/or maintain personal behaviours and characteristics which are as culturally normative as possible' (Anderson et al 1989). These 'norms' have arisen through the identification of a range of normal characteristics of populations gained from the widespread use of surveys. They are therefore based in medical and statistical models that have become part of our social and moral fabric (Moser 2000). Normal characteristics are determined from the statistically most common or usual occurrence of particular phenomenon in particular samples of a population (Armstrong 1987). When a person fails to demonstrate an expected norm they become viewed as abnormal, demonstrating a failure to adopt the subject positions prescribed for them. Responses to the failure of people to meet norms can be to blame them for their 'abnormal' characteristics and expect them to restore the 'norms' in their life.

Chronically ill people fall outside the expected norms by their failure to restore themselves to 'normal' health. However, whilst they are viewed as 'abnormal', once diagnosed with a chronic illness, a different set of norms emerge that are identified as acceptable characteristics within their illness state. For example, people with End Stage Renal Disease (ESRD) are unable to maintain a 'normal' biochemical state due to the loss of renal function. A different set of biochemical values is then considered normal for this group of patients. Surveillance becomes an important strategy for health care workers to monitor patient compliance with these expected norms through regular screening (in ESRD this involves regular monitoring of serum sodium and potassium levels).

### Stigma

One consequence of viewing chronic illnesses within discourses of normalisation and individualism is the experience of stigma. According to Carr & Halpin (2002, p 1):

> The word 'stigma' means a mark or sign of disgrace or discredit, and 'to stigmatise' means to regard a person as unworthy or disgraceful. The consequences of being regarded in such a way include shame, humiliation, ostracism and despair.

The influential work of Goffman (1963) has the potential to guide current understandings of stigma. He identified three main types of stigma: physical deformity, character blemishes and tribal stigma within chronic illness.

The stigma of physical deformity occurs when there is a difference between the expected norm of perfect physical condition and the actual physical condition (Lubkin & Larsen 2002). Many chronic illnesses result in some degree of physical change or deformity that is identified as not 'normal' by other members of society who do not possess that trait. This identification sets the person apart; for example, the altered mobility related to rheumatoid arthritis and Parkinson's disease.

Character blemishes provoke the second type of stigma described by Goffman (1963). There is a moral element to this type of stigma, as character blemishes are associated with traits such as dishonesty, addiction, mental illness, and lack of control (Lubkin & Larsen 2002). Gray (1999) described HIV/AIDS as 'both life threatening and often viewed as an illness associated with socially inappropriate or undesirable behaviours' (p 39). Consequently, the stigma associated with a diagnosis of HIV/AIDS occurs when other members of society form a judgment that holds the person who has HIV/AIDS accountable for their behaviour in contracting the illness, in a way that might be described as 'blaming the victim'.

Tribal stigma or prejudice, the third of Goffman's observations, occurs where there are differences between group identity on the basis of religion, race, nationality and beliefs. An extreme example of tribal stigma was shown during the Second World War when the Nazi regime demonstrated intolerance and prejudice toward Jews resulting in the large-scale murders of the Holocaust (Doosje & Branscombe 2003).

Building on Goffman's work, Jones and colleagues (1984) identified six dimensions that influence interpersonal relationships and the degree of stigmatisation experienced:

1. *concealability* refers to the degree of visibility of the variance from 'normal';

2. *course* of the condition reflects the extent to which the condition changes over time and any associated incapacity;

3. *strain* relates to the stress that the stigma places on interpersonal relationships, whereby the greater the visibility, the more relationships are strained;

4. *aesthetic* qualities refers to the degree that the presentation of the condition is perceived as unattractive;

5. *cause* relates to how the identified origin of the condition can influence the stigma experienced; for example, if the disease is perceived as contagious, or acquired through unacceptable behaviour rather than congenital; and

6. *peril* focuses on the perceived dangers associated with stigmatised persons. Fear of dangerous behaviour associated with mental illness is common.

Using these features, different diseases can be distinguished as discredited or discreditable (Goffman 1963). Disorders where features cannot be hidden are discredited (for example, the skin disease of psoriasis), are discredited because of the visible difference between those with and those without the condition. The affected person is viewed as discredited from the 'norm'. Where features of a disorder can be hidden allowing the person to 'pass as normal' the disease is viewed as discreditable, as the person has the potential to become discredited (Joachim & Acorn 2000). Joanne, with a diagnosis of Type 1 diabetes, was able to 'pass as normal', but was caught in the hiding of her disease and subsequently became 'discredited'.

Given this understanding of how stigma can arise, the issue of disclosure is important. The decision to disclose an illness to others is influenced, in part, by the perception of the level of stigma likely to be encountered and the visibility of the disease (Joachim & Acorn 2000, Scambler 1998). Where the disease is not visible, the possible risk associated with disclosure is the threat of being stigmatised and therefore discredited.

There has been considerable research exploring stigma and disclosure in a range of different diseases. Comparison across these studies is limited due to different definitions of stigma and disclosure but there appears to be two contrasting findings related to the risks and benefits of disclosure (Comer et al 1999). The first is that disclosure enhances mental health and mobilises community and family support. The second approach is that disclosure induces stigmatisation and is accompanied by poor mental health (Comer et al 1999). This creates a real challenge for nurses, who must decide whether to encourage people with an illness to share their experiences with others in the hope of receiving social support, or suggest that the illness be kept secret, to avoid stigma and its outcomes.

These challenges confronting people with chronic illness frequently lead to non-disclosure. Goffman (1963) identified covering and passing as strategies used by people to minimise their experiences of stigma. 'Covering' a visible chronic illness involves acknowledging the condition whilst attempting to decrease the anxiety and stress experienced by those who do not have it (Joachim & Acorn 2000). Joking about a defect is an example of covering. It is an attempt to make 'normals' feel comfortable. Covering enables individuals with stigmatised conditions to fit in with 'normals' as well as with the group being stigmatised. For example, a Melbourne comedian, Steady Eddie, has cerebral palsy and uses humour about his condition to make people comfortable.

Alternatively, passing is a strategy to conceal and keep the condition secret, to attempt to pass as 'normal' (Goffman 1963). Joachim & Acorn (2000, p 245) following Goffman (1963) confirm that passing 'involves deliberate concealment, and differs from covering, where the intent is to downplay a condition'. A major objective of passing behaviour is to fit in with the 'normal' group and strategies to achieve this objective include eradicating all signs of the condition, assigning the signs of the condition to other less stigmatising illnesses and dividing the world into those people who know and those who do not know about the condition. According to Joachim & Acorn (2000) a person effectively passes when they are either accepted as part of the normal group or are caught out in the deception (for example, if the person with diabetes has a serious hypoglycaemic event). Passing is a source of stress because of the constant worry associated with the possibility of discovery (Thorn 1993).

# Challenges for nursing practice

This chapter has argued that the medically produced view of chronic illness has become the foundation for most investigations of chronic illness, and that this has significant consequences for those with chronic illness, their families, health care workers and society. There has been a continuation of a predominantly narrow and paternalistic approach toward chronically ill people. Chronically ill people have become implicated as responsible for their illness and their experiences of illness have been objectified by scientific investigation.

The dominance of scientific approaches as the basis for understanding chronic illness has limited investigations to an exploration of the way illness occurs in individuals. The 'person' (not the individual) with chronic illness has been isolated from scientific investigations and, as a consequence, families and the social outcomes of long-term illness have been minimised or frequently ignored. However, there is a growing challenge to the dominance of 'biomedical' views. People with disability are among those who are demanding that difference become 'a source of celebration rather than a rationale for rejection' (Scrambler 1998, p 1054).

Nurses need to examine their practices to identify how they support the use of 'idealised norms' in attempting to facilitate the rehabilitation and ongoing care of people with chronic illness. The foundations of these 'norms' remain uncontested while nurses, and other health care professionals, continue to endorse the dominant constructions of chronic illness. A key strategy to assist in contesting the effects of normalisation is to engage in partnership with people with chronic illness. Chapter 13 of this text, Empowering Partnerships: Nurses and Those They Care For, provides some strategies for achieving this, as well as identifying the benefits of so doing.

Developing meaningful partnerships with client groups has been promoted for some time but is not easy to enact. Effective communication between health care practitioners and patients has been repeatedly acknowledged as one of the significant factors in fostering collaborative relationships, but communication remains identified as ineffective much of the time (for examples see Partridge 2002, Rassmussen, Wellard & Nankurvis 2001, Wellard 2001). The responsibility of nurses is to continue to critically evaluate the strategies they employ to support people with chronic illness and be mindful of the taken-for-granted norms we apply in developing interventions. It is vital that we take the risk of engaging in relationships with patients where we value equality and negotiation as central.

# Conclusion

We have argued that our understandings of chronic illness have been constructed within the discourses (or worldviews) of science, individualism and normalisation. These discourses shape the way we respond to, and support, people with chronic illness.

Biomedical approaches to understanding illness experience focus on the physical body and the variation from 'normal' that occurs. Subsequently psychological and sociological knowledge has built from that 'medicalised' view of the person with a chronic illness. Mapping of disease trajectories, measuring quality of life and compliance with treatment have all been incorporated into health care practices to assist in identifying the ways in which people with chronic illnesses meet the expected progression of their disease and take responsibility for their individual care. The experience of stigma is one of the outcomes of approaching care through identifying people as abnormal if they do not meet the expected norm.

In Joanne's situation, her expressed willingness to comply with the treatment seemed to make a difference to the response of the team involved in managing her illness. As she explained, 'The fact that insulin was failing to control my sugar levels felt as if it were a personal failure of my own—first my pancreas doesn't work properly and now the treatment isn't working either.' The health team could have reassured Joanne that this is not common and she should not feel responsible for this happening, but they were influenced by a view that the unstable sugar levels must be because she was non-compliant with her diet. Once it was recognised that insulin resistance was to blame, things changed. Joanne's case really made her nurse reflect on her own practice:

> It has certainly made me aware that you have to keep an open mind when you are dealing with people who have diabetes or any chronic illness for that matter. Judging and blaming a client for problems associated with their illness does little toward helping them to constructively manage the problems associated with it.

## Tutorial questions

1. Select two common chronic diseases (diabetes, asthma, chronic heart failure or chronic obstructive pulmonary disease (COPD)) and map the possible trajectories that may be experienced.

   a) Identify the pathophysiological features.

   b) What are the psychosocial factors?

   c) Is compliance a concern?

   d) Are there significant variations between the two diseases?

2. What are the accepted 'norms' for a person with asthma?

3. Use Goffman's theory to identify possible sources of stigma for a person with a sexually transmitted infection, such as herpes simplex virus II.

4. What response would you, as a health care professional, give to Joanne when she stated that 'no one seems to be listening to me, or seems to understand that I am following my treatment plan but my blood glucose level is still rising'?

5. Reflect on an instance of stigmatisation you have either experienced or observed. Using Jones et al's (1984) six dimensions, outline how they apply to this situation.

# References

Abercrombie N, Hill S, Turner B 1986 *Sovereign Individuals of Capitalism*. Allen & Unwin, Sydney

Anderson JM, Elfert H, May A, Lai M 1989 Ideology in the clinical context: chronic illness, ethnicity and the discourse of normalisation. *Sociology of Health and Illness* 11(3):253–278

Armstrong D 1987 Theoretical tensions in biopsychosocial medicine. *Social Science and Medicine* 25(11):1213–1218

Australian Institute of Health and Welfare (AIHW) 2002 *Chronic Diseases and Associated Risk Factors in Australia*. AHIW, Canberra

Burckhardt CS, Woods SL, Schultz AA, Ziebarth DM 1989 Quality of life of adults with chronic illness: A psychometric study. *Research in Nursing and Health* 12:347–354

Callaghan WM, Berg CJ 2002 Maternal mortality surveillance in the United States: moving into the twenty-first century'. *Journal American Medical Women's Association* 57(3):131–139

Cameron K, Gregor F 1987 Chronic Illness and compliance. *Journal of Advanced Nursing* 12:671–676

Carr V, Halpin S 2002 Stigma and discrimination, National Survey of Mental Health and Wellbeing Bulletin 6. Publications Production Unit (Governance and Business Strategy Branch), Commonwealth Department of Health and Ageing, Canberra

Comer LK, Henker B, Kemeny M, Wyatt G 1999 Illness disclosure and mental health among women with HIV:AIDS. *Journal of Community and Applied Social Psychology* 10:338–353

Corbin JM, Strauss A 1991 A nursing model for chronic illness management based on the trajectory framework. *Scholarly Inquiry for Nursing Practice* 5:155–174

Cooper MC 1990 Chronic illness and nursing's ethical challenge. *Holistic Nursing Practice* 5(1):10–16

Crawford R 1984 A cultural account of 'health': control, release, and the social body. In: J McKinlay (ed), *Issues in the political economy of health care*. Travistock, New York

Doosje B, Branscombe NR 2003 Attributions for the negative historical actions of a group. *European Journal of Social Psychology* 33(2):235–248

Eddins BR 1985 Chronic self-destructiveness as manifested by noncompliance behavior in the hemodialysis patient. *Journal of Nephrology Nursing* July/August:194–198

Fielding D, Duff A 1999 Compliance with treatment protocols: interventions for children with chronic illness. *Arch Dis Child* (80):196–200

Foucault M 1972 *The Archaeology of Knowledge*. Pantheon Books, New York

Foucault M 1975a, *The Birth of the Clinic: An Archaeology of Medical Perception*. Vintage Books, New York

Foucault M 1975b *Discipline and Punish: The Birth of the Prison*. Pantheon Books, New York

Fries JF, Spitz PW 1990 The Hierarchy of Patient Outcomes. In: B. Spilker (ed), *Quality of Life Assessments in Clinical Trials*. Raven Press, New York

Garratt A, Schmidt L, Mackintosh A, Fitzpatrick R 2002 Quality of life measurement: Bibliographic study of patient assessed health outcomes. *British Medical Journal* 324:1417–1419

Gerhardt U 1990 Qualitative research on chronic illness: the issue and the story. *Social Science and Medicine* 30(11):1149–1159

Glaser BG, Strauss AL 1967 *The Discovery of Grounded Theory: Strategies for Qualitative Research.* Aldine Publishing, New York

Goffman E 1963 *Stigma. Notes on the management of spoiled identity.* Prentice Hall, Englewood Cliffs, New Jersey

Gray JJ 1999 The difficulties of women living with HIV infection. *Journal of Psychosocial Nursing & Mental Health Services* 37(5):39–43

Hailey BJ, Moss SB 2000 Compliance behaviour in patients undergoing haemodialysis: a review of literature. *Psychology, Health & Medicine* 5(4):395–406

Hinman AR 1998 Global progress in infectious disease control. *Vaccine* 16(11–12):1116–1121

Joachim G, Acorn S 2000 Stigma of visible and invisible chronic conditions. *Journal of Advanced Nursing* 32(1):243–248

Jones E, Farina A, Hastorf A, Markus H, Miller DT, Scott RA 1984 *Social Stigma: the Psychology of Marked Relationships.* Freeman, New York

Kelly MP, May D 1982 Good and bad patients: a review of the literature and a theoretical critique. *Journal of Advanced Nursing* 7:147–156

Kontz MM 1989 Compliance redefined and implications for home care. *Holistic Nurse Practice* 3(2):54–64

Kyngäs H 2000 Compliance of adolescents with chronic disease. *Journal of Clinical Nursing* 9:549–556

Kyngäs H, Duffy ME, Kroll T 2000 Conceptual analysis of compliance. *Journal of Clinical Nursing* 9:5–12

Lamping DL, Campbell KA 1990 Hemodialysis Compliance: Assessment, Prediction and Intervention. *Seminars in Dialysis* 3(1):52–56

Lowenberg JS 1995 Health promotion and the 'ideology of choice'. *Public Health Nursing* 12(5):319–323

Lubkin IM 1998 *Chronic Illness: Impact and Interventions,* 4th edn. Jones and Bartlett, Boston

Lubkin I, Larsen P 2002 *Chronic Illness: Impact and Interventions,* 5th edn. Jones and Bartlett Publishers, Sudbury, Massachusetts

Molzahn AE, Northcott HC, Dossetor JB 1997 Quality of life of individuals with end stage renal disease: perceptions of patients, nurse and physicians. *ANNA Journal* 24(3):325–335

Moser I 2000 Against normalisation: subverting norms of ability and disability. *Science as Culture* 9(2):201–240

O'Connor DB, Shimizu M 2002 Sense of personal control, stress and coping style: a cross-cultural study. *Stress and Health* 18:173–183

Partridge MR 2002 Living with a variable disease. *Pulmonary Pharmacology & Therapeutics* 15(6):491–497

Rasmussen B, Wellard SJ, Nankervis A 2001 Consumer issues in navigating health care services for type 1 diabetes. *Journal of Clinical Nursing* 10(5):628–634

Register C 1987 *Living With Chronic Illness: Days of Patience and Passion.* The Free Press, New York

Rolland JS 1987 Chronic Illness and the life cycle: A conceptual framework. *Family Process* 26:203–211

Sanders C, Egger M, Donovan J, Tallon D, Frankel S 1998 Reporting on quality of life in randomized controlled trials: bibliographic study. *British Medical Journal* 317:1191–1194

Scrambler G 1998 Stigma and disease: changing paradigms. *The Lancet* 352:1054–1055

Strauss AL (ed) 1984 *Where Medicine Fails.* Transaction, New Brunswick

Strauss AL, Corbin J, Fagerhaugh S, Glaser BG, Maines D, Suczek B, Wiener, CL 1984 *Chronic Illness and the Quality of Life.* Mosby, St Louis

Tanenberg RJ 2001 The'non-compliant' patient. *Diabetes Forecast* February:11

Tesh SN 1990 *Hidden Arguments: Political Ideology and Disease Prevention Policy.* Rutgers University Press, New Brunswick

Thorne SE 1990 Constructive noncompliance in chronic illness. *Holistic Nurse Practice* 5(1):62–69

Turk DC, Kerns RD 1985 *Health, Illness and Families: A Life-Span Perspective.* John Wiley & Sons, New York

Turk D, Rudy T E 1991 Neglected topics in the treatment of chronic pain patients—relapse, non-compliance, and adherence enhancement. *Pain* 44:5–28

Vermeire E, Hearnshaw H, Van Royen P, Denekens J 2001 Patient adherence to treatment: three decades of research. A comprehensive review. *Journal of Clinical Pharmacy and Therapeutics* 26:331–342

Wellard SJ, Rushton C 2002 Influences of spatial practices on pressure ulcer management in the context of spinal cord injury. *International Journal of Nursing Practice* 8:221–227

Wellard SJ, Street AF 1999 Family Issues in Home Based Care. *International Journal of Nursing Practice.* 5:132–136

Wellard SJ 2001 Mapping the management of pressure sores in SCI: an Australian case study. *SCI Nursing,* 18(1):11–18

# Chapter 9

## Psychosocial Aspects of Pain and Fatigue

*Alexandra McCarthy*

**This chapter discusses:**

- the psychosocial issues associated with pain and fatigue in chronic illness;
- the characteristics of pain and fatigue;
- issues to consider in the assessment of pain and fatigue;
- the ways that pain, fatigue, anxiety, depression and sleep dysfunction are inter-related in chronic illness; and
- interventions to improve the psychosocial outcomes of clients who experience pain and fatigue associated with chronic illness.

The purpose of this chapter is to give you an insight into the psychosocial dimension of the pain and fatigue that are often associated with chronic illnesses. Rheumatoid arthritis is a typical example of a lifelong and lifechanging condition that is usually accompanied by pain and fatigue. For example, all people who have flare-ups of rheumatoid arthritis experience acute pain, and some degree of chronic pain is reported in as many as 83% of all rheumatoid arthritis clients (Stone et al 1997). Similarly, between 33% and 100% of people with rheumatoid arthritis report a consistent lack of energy, with more than one-third displaying significant levels of fatigue (Crosby 1991, Belza 1995, Wolfe et al 1996, Stone et al 1997, Fifield et al 1998). A case study of rheumatoid arthritis will serve as our example in this chapter. It will demonstrate the complexity of the relationship between the physiological, psychological and sociological variables that influence pain and fatigue, and how this complexity must be appreciated in order for us to care for our clients well.

# Case study

Fiona, is a 45-year-old professional woman, who is married with two children under the age of 10 years. Fiona was diagnosed with rheumatoid arthritis by her GP and, after she continued to report increasing joint pain, stiffness and continual tiredness, the GP referred her to a specialist for more intensive management. Fiona's story, an excerpt of which follows, is very typical of people who experience rheumatoid arthritis.

'I remember I was so anxious about what the specialist would say—I thought he might think I was malingering or something. I wondered whether he would believe me, about how incredibly tired and down I was all the time, and how much the pain and stiffness got in the way of my work and doing even normal things at home. At home I'd get teary because my husband and kids had to take on more and more of the jobs around the house and it was causing a few arguments. I was really anxious about how it was affecting my performance at work and I was very worried that I'd get the sack if I took too many days off. I was really busy at work, pretty overloaded, and even I thought that all that was wrong with me was a bit of stress ...

... I really thought the specialist would just give me a script for an antidepressant to cheer me up and a sleeping pill to get me off to sleep at night. I had no idea that he would tell me what I had was forever, and that it would get worse from time to time, and that the whole family would have to make adjustments for my rheumatoid arthritis. And he gave me a pile of scripts for pain medication and pills to stop my joints flaring up all the time, and a referral to an occupational therapist for splints, and to a physiotherapist for exercises. All I could think about was how am I going to manage all that plus what I have to do already when I'm feeling so awful?'

Fiona's story illustrates very clearly the close relationship between physiological variables like pain and fatigue and the psychosocial context in which they occur. It demonstrates that while it is important to identify and treat the physical causes of chronic illnesses like rheumatoid arthritis, we also need to look at the ways that chronic pain and fatigue also affect the client's long-term lifestyle choices, their family and working life, and their emotions. We also need to be aware that the psychosocial aspects of pain and fatigue have the potential to affect the person's physical health outcomes in a circular fashion. This is because they affect a person's ability to perform their normal activities of daily living, such as maintaining the exercise and diet programs that help prevent ill health.

As you work through this chapter, you will come to understand that the physiological and the psychosocial aspects of chronic pain and fatigue are so closely linked that if we address only one aspect while ignoring the other, then our efforts to help the client will probably be ineffective. We need to understand what pain and fatigue are, and then the different elements that contribute to pain and fatigue in chronic illnesses, before we can identify appropriate interventions for care.

We'll begin with a brief overview of the physiological cause of Fiona's pain and fatigue, and look at how it influences the larger psychosocial picture. Then we'll look at the way that the psychosocial aspects of disease in turn influence her physical health outcomes.

# Pain

This section will explore the physiological bases of pain and fatigue and then review definitions and characteristics of pain and how to assess the pain a person is experiencing.

## The cause of pain and fatigue in rheumatoid arthritis

Rheumatoid arthritis develops when the immune system, for reasons unknown, becomes dysfunctional. The immune impairment usually results in inflammation of the joints, but other connective tissues, such as blood vessels and the linings of the heart and lungs, can also become inflamed. Because it is mainly the structure of the joints that is disturbed, rheumatoid arthritis results in progressive swelling, contraction, and deformity of these areas. The inflammation can cause a great deal of pain and stiffness, particularly in the joints. Joint stiffness also means the person cannot move as freely, leading to the muscle wasting that often underlies the development of fatigue.

Unfortunately, while pain and fatigue are common symptoms of rheumatoid arthritis, they can be very difficult for nurses to isolate, measure and assess. For example, we cannot *see* pain or fatigue. There is also debate as to what pain and fatigue actually are, because pain and fatigue are so dependent on the description and interpretation of the person who experiences them. These difficulties are further complicated by the nature of the pain and fatigue in rheumatoid arthritis, which fluctuates between acute, chronic, and remission phases over the course of the illness. Similarly, clients who are in the same stage of the illness may experience pain and fatigue very differently, with some severely affected and others barely noticing it. There are some consistencies across these symptoms, however, that enable us to arrive at definitions that are useful in psychosocial assessments.

## Definitions and characteristics of pain

Definitions of pain vary from the strictly physiological to those that reflect a more holistic worldview. One of the most useful definitions of pain was proposed by the International Association for the Study of Pain (IASP 1979, p 242):

> Pain is an unpleasant sensory and emotional experience associated with actual or potential tissue damage, or described in terms of such damage. Pain is always subjective.

This is expressed more simply by McCaffery & Beebe (1994), who propose that pain is whatever the person who experiences it says it is, occurring whenever that person says it does.

**116**

These definitions are useful within the psychosocial context because they incorporate factors other than the purely physiological that contribute to pain. That is, the role played by psychosocial factors, such as emotions and the events happening in the person's life at the time, is accounted for. These definitions are also useful because:

- Pain is always assumed to be subjective, meaning that one person's experience of pain is not necessarily the same as another person's, but it is pain nonetheless.

- Experience of pain is acknowledged to be different between individuals—that what may trigger severe pain in one person may only mildly affect another.

- It is assumed that a person is in pain if they say they are, and a person's experience of pain must not be denied.

## Pain assessment

Based on these holistic definitions of pain, a thorough pain assessment that is grounded in the client's description is extremely important. An important first step in pain assessment is to differentiate chronic pain from acute pain, which has different origins and different treatments.

Acute pain is usually caused by an obvious injury or illness. It tends to have a defined onset and lasts for a certain period of time, and is easy to treat in comparison with chronic pain. In rheumatoid arthritis, for example, flare-ups of the condition will cause an acute pain that is relatively easy to relieve with anti-inflammatory and pain medication. Acute pain is also identified by its effects on the sympathetic nervous system, so that clients become anxious, with a raised blood pressure and pulse rate. These very obvious symptoms of injury, raised pulse and blood pressure tend to prejudice people's views of what the person in pain should look like. As a result, most people think that people complaining of pain should have an obvious injury or cause for their pain, and show definite signs such as grimacing that demonstrate it. This is often not the case with chronic pain.

In contrast to acute pain, it is often not easy to determine exactly when and why chronic pain begins. More often than not, it has a subtle onset that is difficult for the client to pinpoint. In general, chronic pain begins as a response to long-term disease processes. It is usually present for longer than six months before it is diagnosed as chronic. Unfortunately, the difficulty in ascertaining a definite cause for chronic pain, and the way it tends to linger, may elicit a lot less understanding from other people (including nurses) even when a person is definitely known to have a condition that can cause pain. For example, people with chronic pain may appear depressed and lethargic and, therefore, they can be difficult to relate to if you do not know them well. Furthermore, because they have become so accustomed to the presence of pain, there is little reflex stimulation of the sympathetic nervous system. This means that people with chronic pain rarely display the 'obvious' symptoms of pain such as grimacing, or raised heart rate and blood pressure. In fact, their physical signs are usually quite normal, and this may prejudice others into thinking they have no pain at all. Chronic pain is just as debilitating as acute pain, however, and should be taken just as seriously.

# Fatigue

This section will explore definitions and characteristics of fatigue as well as how to assess for fatigue.

## Definitions and characteristics of fatigue

Like pain, fatigue is also hard to define and assess, as it is such a subjective experience. Nurses, who are trained to make judgements on the basis of what they can actually see and measure, are not readily able to do so with fatigue and are therefore generally reliant on the client's description of the experience. Unfortunately, the way the nurse actually interprets the client's description of their fatigue is not necessarily an accurate reflection of what the person is really experiencing. The factors that might colour the nurse's interpretation include the quality of education they have received about fatigue themselves and the way they have been socialised to think about fatigue.

However, our understanding of fatigue is gradually improving with a more holistic focus. One of the best definitions of fatigue identifies it as a subjective feeling of tiredness, that may or may not be related to activity, which becomes problematic in chronic illness because it leads to disruption of daily activities and cannot be relieved by rest (Fishbain et al 2003). Like our definitions of pain, this definition recognises the subjective rather than objective nature of fatigue. This definition also incorporates the difficulties that fatigue causes in daily life; and that it is what the person experiencing says it is.

## Fatigue assessment

People with rheumatoid arthritis generally experience both acute and chronic fatigue through the course of their illness. Like the experiences of acute and chronic pain, the experience of acute fatigue is different to that of chronic fatigue. It is important to differentiate whether fatigue is acute or chronic, as they often have a different origin and different effects on the client and, therefore, different treatments.

Acute fatigue is episodic in nature, with a rapid onset and a quick resolution. In rheumatoid arthritis clients, acute fatigue is generally associated with obvious triggers such as over-exertion or flare-ups of the disease that result in increased joint pain. Acute fatigue can often be successfully and rapidly relieved with anti-inflammatory medication and rest. In contrast, similar to chronic pain, it is difficult to pinpoint a cause for chronic fatigue and it may not even be related to the person's activity level. The chronic fatigue produced by illnesses such as rheumatoid arthritis is a persistent, cumulative sensation not relieved by resting. In fact, rest can exacerbate chronic fatigue. Chronic fatigue also has a significant psychosocial component, so both these factors must be addressed for it to be relieved (Crosby 1991, Belza 1995, Wolfe et al 1996, Barsky et al 1999).

# The pain/fatigue complex in chronic illness

Consistent with the definitions of acute and chronic pain and fatigue outlined above, the psychosocial approach to illness views the factors influencing levels of pain and fatigue as numerous and interrelated. There is evidence, for example, that the physical causes of pain in cases like Fiona's include tissue degeneration and joint restriction. Other evidence demonstrates that the physical causes of her fatigue may include progressive muscle weakness and the tiredness that is a common side effect of various medical treatments (Gentile et al 2003). Commonsense would also tell us that these physiological variables interact with each other, for the more severe the pain and the longer it lasts, the greater the chance of developing fatigue (Brandt 1997, Fishbain et al 2003).

However, the physiological variables that contribute to pain and fatigue are also influenced by psychosocial variables in an additive and interactive fashion. This is because the physiological sensations of pain and fatigue have a peripheral, sensory component that is processed centrally in the brain, which then determines our behavioural response. The way the brain processes the sensory components of pain and fatigue is profoundly influenced by (Barsky et al 1999):

- the way we have been socialised to view pain and fatigue;

- our emotional state at the time we experience pain and fatigue; and

- our previous experiences of pain and fatigue.

For example, if Fiona has learnt from her past experience that a flare-up of her joints will lead to pain, she is more likely to become depressed about that flare-up, and her depression may subsequently influence her perception of her pain in a negative way. Similarly, if Fiona has been exposed to work cultures that view taking a 'sickie' for chronic fatigue as malingering, she will be anxious not to take time off to prove her work ethic. She will then strive to work harder despite her tiredness, ending up more tired than ever—and possibly cause a flare-up of her condition that will result in even more pain and fatigue.

The physiological variables contributing to pain and fatigue not only influence each other but can be a cause and effect of pain and fatigue as well. We can see that a physiological factor like pain can result in the psychosocial factor of depression and that, in turn, depression can influence pain. Similarly, the psychosocial variable of cultural anxiety can contribute to the physiological variable of fatigue, and fatigue in turn can influence the level of anxiety. The additive and interactive nature of this process highlights how closely interconnected chronic illness, pain, fatigue, emotional disturbances and social disruption are. Fiona's case history is a good example of how a combination of the chronic disease process, the demanding treatment regimes, the psychological adjustments, the alteration of social roles, and the views of significant others within the person's social context are part of a complex of factors that contribute to the person's experience of pain and fatigue (Belza 1995, Brandt 1997, Schuman 1997, Strahl et al 2000, Sinclair 2001, Barlow et al 2002; Gentile et al 2003). The following discussion will tease out three major psychosocial components of pain and fatigue, and the ways that one variable can sustain another to produce chronic pain and fatigue. These variables are anxiety, depression, and sleep disturbance.

## Anxiety

Anxiety is an unpleasant state that is associated with feelings of uneasiness, apprehension, and heightened physiological arousal, such as increased heart rate and blood pressure (Plotnik 2002). Fiona's story reveals her valid concern that a worsening of her illness has the potential to profoundly affect her quality of life. This anxiety is typical of people with rheumatoid arthritis who have experienced a great deal of pain (Neville et al 1999). Research indicates that nearly 50% of rheumatoid arthritis clients are at risk of developing clinical anxiety, and that this anticipatory anxiety can worsen the pain experience for them (Barlow et al 1999, Strahl et al 2000). Furthermore, pain-related anxiety can predict other complaints such as fatigue (Brandt 1997, Strahl et al 2000).

Fiona's anxiety is not surprising, given the unpredictable and disruptive nature of her chronic illness and the pain that defines it. An interesting psychosocial explanation of her anxiety is that it is a response to her loss of control over her body (Melanson & Downe-Wamboldt 2003). Our society demands that we have predictable bodily functions, and we also have a personal responsibility for maintaining that function (Turner 1992, Frank 1995, Turner 1996). For example, we are expected to exercise appropriately and keep our weight down to prevent the onset of conditions like arthritis that prevent us from performing our social roles. Unfortunately, our culture also has a contradictory approach to illness that feeds this anxiety and generates a lot of confusion for people with chronic illnesses. On the one hand, people who have adopted a biomedical perspective of illness could argue that Fiona is not responsible for her symptoms in any way, because her pain and fatigue are purely the result of problems within her immune system. On the other hand, it is not uncommon to hear other people, including nurses, attribute the responsibility for illness to the behaviour of the person who has it. Have you ever heard, for example, statements inferring that those who develop chronic illnesses such as heart disease have only themselves to blame because they don't eat well or exercise enough? Or that if they had been more careful with their diet, they wouldn't have become ill in the first place?

Regardless of these contradictory standpoints, society as a whole does expect Fiona to behave in certain ways to legitimise her status as a sick person. For example, she cannot diagnose her own condition—this can only be done by an expert, such as a doctor (Turner 1996). It is not likely that her workmates would remain sympathetic to Fiona's reports of overwhelming fatigue if she hadn't sought a medical explanation for it. In addition, Fiona has certain roles and responsibilities that must be fulfilled when she enters the 'sick role' (Parsons 1950). You will have read about Parsons' theory in Chapter 2 Health, Wellness, Illness, Healing and Holism, and Nursing, and you will see Parson's work discussed again in Chapter 13, Empowering Partnerships: Nurses and Those They Care For.

According to Parsons, the way Fiona meets her 'sick role' responsibilities also determines whether other people accept her in that role or not (Parsons 1950). So, while Fiona is exempt from her usual obligations while she is unwell, she can only continue to be exempt if she is seen to be following the expert's advice in order to become well again. It is not socially desirable to want to be ill, so she is expected to fight her symptoms with a positive attitude, to comply with medical treatment, and to adopt lifestyle changes to prevent the development of further pain and fatigue. Fiona will always be judged by her workmates and acquaintances according to how well she fulfils these responsibilities.

Nurses who operate from the psychosocial perspective may believe it is reasonable for people who experience many episodes of pain and fatigue to naturally have adaptive responses such as mild anxiety. Anxiety would help prepare Fiona for subsequent flare-ups of her disease by keeping her mindful of the need to prevent pain and fatigue from happening again. Unfortunately, the expectation that Fiona will monitor her own illness to prevent further deterioration means that she treads a very fine line indeed, for more than a mild anxiety about pain and fatigue paradoxically can be viewed by some health professionals as taking issues of control too far. Severe anxiety is seen as problematic because it disrupts the person's physiological and psycho-social wellbeing.

People who are considered more than healthily mindful of their symptoms tend to be labelled as hypochondriacs or somatisers. Somatisation is the tendency to report symptoms that cannot be adequately explained (or understood) by the health care team. A person with an amplified somatic style is described as one who reports that their experience of bodily sensations, including chronic pain and chronic fatigue, are noxious and worrisome, and considers them signs of serious disease even when medical opinion does not consider them pathological (Barsky et al 1999). It is apparently characteristic of this 'style' of managing one's illness that clients are hyper-vigilant and preoccupied with their bodily sensations, reacting to their sensations of pain and fatigue with thinking and behaviour that make the symptoms seem worse than the health professional believes they are.

Whatever your thoughts about the labelling of people as hypochondriacs in this way, it is clear from the research that severe anxiety about the possibility of pain does result in more frequent experiences of pain (Barsky 1999).

## Depression

Depression is described as a loss of interest or pleasure in nearly all activities and is usually accompanied by one or more of the following symptoms: changes in weight or appetite, sleep disruption, lack of concentration and energy, and feelings of guilt or worthlessness (Bailey et al 2002). Fiona's story reveals that she has typical signs of mild depression. But it is difficult to discern what came first—her pain, her fatigue or her depression—because the depression that often accompanies chronic illnesses can modulate the perception of pain and fatigue. For example, the severity of the fatigue reported by rheumatoid arthritis clients is related to their depression levels at the time; and depressive symptoms frequently coincide with reports of greater pain and inability to cope with the normal activities of daily living (Brandt 1997, Fifield et al 1998).

## Living with Illness

Whether depression is a cause or effect of pain and fatigue, at least 32% of rheumatoid arthritis clients are at risk of developing clinical depression (Barlow et al 1999). The additive and interactive nature of the pain/fatigue complex is also demonstrated in the way that emotional states, especially depression, can impair the function of the immune system (Dobkin and da Costa 2000). As immune dysfunction is the physiological trigger of rheumatoid arthritis, it is evident that people who have rheumatoid arthritis are at the mercy of a vicious cycle of physiological and psychosocial symptoms.

The sociologist Arthur Frank has offered us some insight into the depression that is associated with chronic pain and fatigue (Frank 1995). He argued that depression is a problem in our western society because we view it as a lack of desire to 'live well'. A depressed person who sees only the negatives in their situation is one who lacks gusto for life, who fails to seek new experiences, or to covet new things—which are all activities that mark us as worthwhile individuals in our consumer-oriented culture. A person like Fiona who is depressed, tired and in pain, is viewed as a burden, one who cannot contribute to a society fuelled by desire and the seeking of pleasure. One only has to look at newspaper and magazine articles praising the zest for life shown by certain celebrities in their 'brave battles' against illness and pain to realise that Frank's arguments do apply to our Australian cultural norms.

It is evident that depression in any form is capable of disrupting a person's quality of life, and that life-threatening depression associated with pain and fatigue requires urgent intervention. But some of the labels given by nurses to depressed people, particularly women, could have serious consequences for their future treatment if they are used carelessly. I have already discussed the label of hypochondriasis, which has very negative connotations. An equally disturbing one in the context of depression is 'pain catastrophising', which is often applied to women with rheumatoid arthritis.

Pain catastrophising is an extremely pessimistic appraisal of painful stimuli in rheumatoid arthritis clients. It is a negative view which colours perceptions of other life events and ensures anticipation of a worst-case scenario when there is the slightest twinge of pain (Sinclair 2001). Women in this situation are characterised as personally inadequate and incompetent, obsessed with their symptoms, and prone to exaggerating their pain (Davey & Levy 1998, Shapiro & Astin 1998). While it is seen as a form of cognitive distortion rather than clinical depression, pain catastrophising does share many of the features of depression, and great care must be taken to differentiate between them when assessing clients. It is obviously very important to undertake a full psychosocial assessment and come to defensible conclusions about a client's mental state when you think a client is exaggerating their pain or is obsessed with it. Patients may be attributed labels such as hypochondriac and catastrophiser for the duration of their illness, and this will profoundly influence the way that other nurses will approach their care. Such labelling is at odds with McCaffery and Beebe's commonly accepted definition of pain as whatever the person who experiences it says it is (1994). There are some similarities here with Joanne's story in Chapter 8, Constructions of Chronic Illness. Joanne was not believed when she stated that she was adhering to her recommended treatment regimen for diabetes. In this instance, we see evidence of health professionals believing that they 'know best' what is happening to their patients.

## Altered patterns of sleep

Sleep has a restorative function, promoting health and general wellbeing. Poor quality sleep results in autonomic nervous system and immune impairment, and can culminate in reduced resistance to other stressors and poor quality of life (Edell-Gustafssonet al 2003). Pain and fatigue are often accompanied by disrupted sleep patterns; and poor quality sleep significantly influences the experience of pain, fatigue, anxiety and depression (Crosby 1991, Stone et al 1997, Cohen et al 2000, Edell-Gustafsson et al 2003). For example, between 50% and 70% of people with chronic pain syndromes report sleep difficulties such as frequent waking, decreased length of sleep, daytime tiredness, and non-restorative sleep; and most surveys demonstrate an adverse relationship between chronic fatigue and sleep disturbance (Cohen et al 2000, Gentile et al 2003).

Similar to all the other variables associated with pain and fatigue, it is not clear whether a pre-existing sleep disorder triggers the development of pain and fatigue, or whether the sleep disorder is the result of the pain and fatigue (Stone et al 1997, Fishbain et al 2003). When you think about it though, not being able to sleep when you have an illness is a sensible adaptive response by the body. Pain and fatigue protect us from further injury, and our natural survival instincts ensure the brain is as active as possible when we are unwell so that we remain alert to any further threat—resulting in disturbed sleep patterns (Cohen et al 2000).

People like Fiona who are constantly tired disturb their natural circadian sleep cycle. In response to her fatigue, Fiona may spend increasing amounts of time dozing through the daytime, which in turn triggers frequent awakening during the night. In consequence, her inherent physiological rhythm of sleep is disrupted (Cohen et al 2000). Unfortunately, it seems that once sleep disturbance becomes chronic in this way, treating the underlying pain, anxiety, or depression associated with it may not necessarily resolve the sleep problems. It appears that disruption of the sleep cycle may become self-sustaining, because once a disruptive pattern is established, it becomes programmed into the central nervous system and becomes independent of the symptoms that triggered it in the first place (Lavie et al 1991). However, if the sleep disorder is caught early enough and proves treatable, it is possible to decrease the problems of pain and fatigue (Cohen et al 2000).

# Interventions

After experiencing these symptoms for some time with no relief, Fiona realised she was not coping and consulted her rheumatologist again. We'll conclude with another excerpt from her case study, and discuss the interventions that may assist her in managing the pain and fatigue associated with her chronic illness.

## Case study . . . *continued*

'I'm glad I swallowed my pride and went back to see him. I was lucky, because he understood how bad I was feeling and how this illness was just taking over my life. He wrote me a different script for pain relief; he organised for me to go to counselling, and referred me to a self-help group and to a sleep disorder clinic. It's early days yet, but at least I feel I can get some sort of control over my arthritis, which is half the battle for me.'

The treatment of the pain and fatigue related to chronic illness would make a book in itself and it can only be examined briefly here. In general, the psychosocial approach to helping Fiona with her pain and fatigue may include the strategies discussed below.

## Attention to her subjective description of her symptoms

The commitment of nurses to long-term therapy with the client, and an empathetic approach, are necessary when dealing with chronic pain and fatigue, where there is minimal likelihood of complete relief. It is particularly useful to learn how to interpret the client's perspective of their pain and fatigue. Pain and fatigue have meaning to the person who experiences them. To understand their meaning is to understand how they affect the person, which in turn facilitates the delivery of better care (Kleinmann 1988, Melanson & Downe-Wamboldt 2003).

## Psychosocial Interventions

Psychosocial interventions usually include helping clients to take control by teaching them problem solving skills and coping strategies to manage their pain and fatigue. They also involve working through bereavement issues regarding the loss of a fully healthy, physically resilient self and re-negotiating relationships with friends, family, employers and colleagues. Chapter 10, Living with Loss and Grief, provides some very useful strategies for assisting people with pain and fatigue to do just that. Addressing the impact of emotions and thoughts on the physical and behavioural dimensions of pain is also important. An overall focus of therapy is the rebuilding of quality of life in the presence of pain and fatigue, where these symptoms are monitored, acknowledged and managed, but not the dominant focus of life (Cohen et al 2000). Cognitive behavioural therapy and group therapy appear to be particularly successful psychosocial interventions (JBIEBNM 1999, Dobkin & da Costa 2000).

While it is important to be aware of the relationship between current symptoms of depression and the client's reports of pain, it is also important to look beyond their current depression to the client's overall history of affective disorders. Even if a client is not clinically depressed at the time they report their pain, those with a previous history of depression are believed to be at risk for more intense levels of pain, and therefore, fatigue (Fifield et al 1998). The thought-restructuring techniques used in cognitive behavioural therapy have a good record of success when used to treat depression related to pain.

## Medication

An understanding of the many drugs used in the treatment chronic illness is vital (Cohen et al 2000). For example, fatigue that is the result of analgesia will limit the amount of treatment an individual is willing to tolerate (Gentile et al 2003). Medication to treat the pain and fatigue should be adjusted after assessing the clients' daily patterns of pain and fatigue. For example, clients whose pain is worse in the mornings may benefit from an increased morning dosage of pain relief, and those with increased fatigue levels in the afternoon and evening may benefit from an altered medication regimen (Stone et al 1997).

## Exercise

While rest is the treatment of choice in cases of acute fatigue to repair injury, gentle exercise is recommended for chronic fatigue. All clients should be encouraged to avoid the over-exertion that can induce acute pain and fatigue. They should also be encouraged to balance rest with graded exercise that improves their energy levels and their sense of wellbeing, and which can modify the perception of pain and fatigue. They should also be encouraged to set realistic goals and aim to ensure that the energy that is available to them is used for appropriate activities.

## Sleep

If it is not treated early, sleep dysfunction can become progressively more difficult to reverse (Cohen et al 2000). Nurses should therefore assess for sleep dysfunction when pain is a problem for clients (Cohen et al 2000). Assessment should include the identification of the extent to which a client's sleep disturbances are in conflict with their expectations of sleep, and their attitudes and beliefs about sleep. Good sleep hygiene can also be taught; for example, the value of a regular routine, keeping afternoon naps short, and the use of a de-activating period of rest and relaxation before going to bed. If the pain that disturbs sleep is treated when the sleep problem first appears, there is a good chance that permanent disruption of the circadian cycle will not ensue.

## Education

Education about the causes and management of pain and fatigue may give a sense of control to the client that improves their psychosocial wellbeing. Clients could be encouraged to read relevant books and access appropriate Internet resources. Joining a support group may be invaluable, since others with the same difficulties can often provide practical strategies for managing pain and fatigue.

# Conclusion

This chapter has given you an insight into the overwhelming and complex nature of pain and fatigue, and the way they are so closely related to the psychosocial context in which they occur. It is important to understand the psychosocial as well as physical implications of these symptoms, as they have the potential to affect every aspect of the client's wellbeing. If you take one thing from reading this chapter, I hope that it is the understanding that if pain and fatigue are not addressed in all the domains of health, then our efforts to help clients manage them will be ineffective.

## Tutorial questions

1.  Identify some strategies which clients experiencing chronic pain may be able to adopt to manage their pain. How might you teach these to the client?

2.  Identify some strategies which clients experiencing chronic fatigue may be able to adopt to maximise their energy levels. How might you teach these to the client?

3.  Our personal beliefs about pain and fatigue profoundly influence the way we approach clients who report these symptoms. What are your beliefs about these symptoms and, if you were confronted with a client who you believed was a 'hypochondriac' or 'catastrophiser', what would you do?

4.  There are many non-invasive pain relief measures available that also address the psychosocial dimensions of pain. What non-invasive or non-pharmaceutical pain relief measures are you aware of, and how might you introduce them to your client and fellow health professionals?

## References

Bailey K P, CD Sauer, Herrell C 2002 Mood disorders. In: MA Boyd (ed), *Psychiatric Nursing: Contemporary Practice*, Lippincott, Philadelphia

Barlow JH, Cullen LA, Rowe IF 1999 Comparison of knowledge and psychological well-being between patients with a short disease duration and patients with more established rheumatoid arthritis. *Patient Education and Counselling* 28:195–203

Barlow JH, Cullen LA, Rowe IF 2002 Educational preferences, psychological well-being and self-efficacy among people with rheumatoid arthritis. *Patient Education and Counselling* 46:11–19

Barsky AJ, Orav J, Ahern DK, Rogers MP 1999 Somatic style and symptom reporting in rheumatoid arthritis. *Psychosomatics* 40(5):396–401

Belza BL 1995 Comparison of self-reported fatigue in rheumatoid arthritis and controls, *Journal of Rheumatology*. 22:639–643

Brandt JC 1997 The relationship of psychobiological parameters to fatigue in patients with rheumatoid arthritis. Dissertation Abstracts International: Section B *The Sciences and Engineering* 57(10-B):6639

Cohen MJM, Menefee LA, Doghranj IK 2000 Sleep in chronic pain problems and treatments. *International Revue of Psychiatry* 12:115–126

Crosby LJ 1991 Factors which contribute to fatigue associated with rheumatoid arthritis. *Journal of Advanced Nursing* 16:974–981

Davey GC, Levy S 1998 Internal statements associated with catastrophic worrying. *Personality and Individual Differences* 26(1):21–32

Dobkin PL, da Costa D 2000 Group psychotherapy for medical patients. *Psychology, Health and Medicine* 5(1):87–94

Edell-Gustafsson UM, Gustavson G, Uhlin PY 2003 Effects of sleep loss in men and women with insufficient sleep suffering from chronic disease: a model for supportive nursing care. *International Journal of Nursing Practice* 9:49–59

Fifield J, Tennen H, Reisine S, McQuillan J 1998 Depression and the long-term risk of pain, fatigue, and disability in patients with rheumatoid arthritis. *Arthritis and Rheumatism* 41(10):1851–1857.

Fishbain DA, Cole B, Cutler RB, Lewis J, Rosomoff HL, Rosomoff CS 2003 Is pain fatiguing? A structured evidence-based review. *Pain Medicine* 4(1):51–62

Frank AW 1995 *The Wounded Storyteller: Body, Illness and Ethics.* University of Chicago Press, Chicago

Gentile S, Delaroziere JC, Farre F, Sambuc R, San Marco JL 2003 Validation of the French multidimensional fatigue inventory (MFI 20). *European Journal of Cancer Care* 12:58–64

IASP 1979 IASP Subcommittee on Taxonomy. *Pain* 6:242–240

JBIEBNM 1999 Group and Individual Therapy in the Treatment of Depression. *Best Practice: Evidence Based Practice Information Sheets for Health Professionals* 3,(2):1–6

Kleinmann A 1988 *The Illness Narratives: Suffering, Healing and the Human Condition.* Basic Books, New York

Lavie P, Nahir M, Lorber M, Schars Y, 1991 Nonsteroidal anti-inflammatory drug therapy in rheumatoid arthritis patients. Lack of association between clinical improvement and effects on sleep. *Arthritis and Rheumatism* 34:655–659

McCaffery M., Beebe A 1994 *Pain: Clinical Manual for Nursing Practice.* Mosby, London

Melanson PM, Downe-Wamboldt B 2003 Confronting life with rheumatoid arthritis. *Journal of Advanced Nursing* 42(2):125–133

Neville C, Fortin PR, FitzCharles M 1999 The needs of patients with arthritis: the patient's perspective. *Arthritis Care and Research* 12(2):85–95

Parsons T 1950 *The Social System.* The Free Press, New York

Plotnik R 2002 *Introduction to Psychology.* Wadsworth-Thomson Learning, California

Schuman CC 1997 Pain and depression as predictors of fatigue in fibromyalgia syndrome patients: an investigation of aggregated and disaggregated data. Dissertation Abstracts International: Section B *The Sciences and Engineering* 57(12-B):7742

Shapiro DH, Astin J 1998 *Control therapy: An integrated approach to psychotherapy, health, and healing.* Wylie, New York

Sinclair, VG 2001 Predictors of pain catastrophizing in women with rheumatoid arthritis. *Archives of Psychiatric Nursing* 15(6):279–288

Stone AA, Broderick JE, Porter LS, Kaell AT 1997 The experience of rheumatoid arthritis pain and fatigue: examining momentary reports and correlates over one week. *Arthritis Care and Research* 10(3):185–193

Strahl CR, Kleinnecht A, Dinnel DL 2000 The role of pain anxiety, coping and pain self-efficacy in rheumatoid arthritis patient functioning. *Behaviour Research and Therapy* 38:863–873

Turner BS 1992 *Regulating Bodies: Essays in Medical Sociology.* Routledge, London

Turner BS 1996 *The Body and Society; Explorations in Social Theory.* Sage Publications, London

Wolfe F, Hawley DJ, Wilson K 1996 The prevalence and meaning of fatigue in rheumatic disease. *Journal of Rheumatology* 23:1407–1417

# Chapter 10

## Living with Loss and Grief

*Cynthia Schultz and Elizabeth Bruce*

**This chapter:**

- demonstrates that loss is an integral part of life;
- describes the impact of loss on individuals in general and, more specifically, those with a chronic condition;
- illustrates how loss can impinge on the family unit;
- encourages reflection on the personal experience of loss;
- defines griefwork and exposes myths about grieving;
- describes the factors influencing individual differences in grieving; and
- presents guidelines for the effective support of those persons who are living with loss and grief, including anticipation of and preparation for, death and dying.

The experience of loss is an inevitable part of life and all significant losses result in grief. Not only do nurses live through their own losses and grief, but often grieve alongside their patients and their families. In an Australian study exploring nurses' perceptions of critical incidents, O'Connor & Jeavons (2003) reported that the nine most stressful incidents for nurses, rated by the sample, were those related to grief. We define grief as the universal and instinctive response to loss, marked by psychological and physical suffering and distress. While grief is a response common to us all, it is also a very individual and personal experience, differing in how it is displayed, and in intensity, impact, and duration. This chapter begins with an examination of loss in life, before delving into its associate—grief. Nerida's story illustrates the impact of loss and grief caused by chronic conditions, such as illness or accident trauma, on the individual and the family. Throughout this chapter, the need for nurses to reflect on personal experiences, as an important step towards understanding and supporting the loss and grief of others, is emphasised. The final section is designed to assist readers to apply loss and grief theories to clinical practice. This section aims to help nurses meet the personal challenges facing them as well as those in their care.

Nerida's story illustrates not only her loss of health, but the associated and subsequent losses and grief experienced by herself, her sister, and her parents. It also illustrates how important it is that the intensity of grief be lessened through acknowledgment and full expression. To fail to allow this opportunity is to invite unspoken sorrow, described so evocatively by Shakespeare (cited in Craig 1943 p 865):

> . . . the grief that does not speak knits up the overwrought heart and bids it break.

## Case study

Nerida was diagnosed with diabetes when she was 5 years of age. At that early age, she could barely begin to contemplate what this diagnosis would mean to her life. But as the years passed, Nerida came to realise more and more just what the diagnosis could mean—loss of a carefree, medication-free existence; missing out on occasions and activities that her sister and her peers enjoyed; being treated as different by her parents, teachers, acquaintances, and thereby losing her sense of normalcy. Also there was the fear and the dread she had sensed early on. This sense had embedded itself in her subconscious thoughts, when as a little girl she had played, sat, and now and then heard her name mentioned during meetings between her parents and the doctors. Her attention hooked onto three words: she could die. How could she have faith in herself or her body, if death was hovering around the corner?

Now 21 years of age, these words and fear of death have retained their drama and have become even more real. She remains terrified of dying, bitterly resentful of being different, of being deemed irresponsible when she does not watch her levels and is rushed to hospital. All her young life, she has been cut off from expressing her grief and her fears, cut off from talking about an intrinsic part of her emotional and physical life. Her grief became submerged by her fears. As a kind of camouflage, her fear and bitterness have been expressed in brazen and cynical behaviour, lashing out at others—especially the nurses and doctors who tend to her during hospitalisation.

## Loss unlimited

Nerida's most obvious loss has been loss of health, but loss occurs in many other forms, many of them not so obvious. One of the most thorough illustrations known to us of the broad spectrum of loss experiences is to be found in the work of Schneider (1984, pp 25–42). He presented more than 70 examples of loss across the lifespan, categorising them as apparent losses, loss as part of change and growth, and competence-related losses.

Examples of apparent losses are:

- loss of relationships through the death of a loved one and/or illness;
- loss of external objects through theft, destruction, disappearance;
- loss of health, youth; and
- environmental loss such as natural disasters, vandalism.

Loss as part of change might be due to:

- divorce, role reversal, breakdown of a relationship;
- moving house, leaving familiar surroundings; and
- changing jobs, retirement.

Unnoticed losses include:

- birth of a child (much joy, but change in lifestyle);
- promotion (cause for celebration, but loss of previous patterns and relationships); and
- shattering of assumptions about fairness, immortality, control.

Schneider (1984) argued that any change has the potential for loss, even those changes which might usually be considered positive in nature. For instance, as a nurse you may at times witness the mixed feelings of patients or clients for whom therapy is about to be terminated due to full recovery. Those persons rejoice over recovery, but may well experience stress and anxiety over the prospect of losing the specialised care and close contact with professional carers to which they have become accustomed, and felt entitled to receive, over an extended period of time.

Finding out about what a change or transition can mean to a patient leads us closer to understanding the conflict between feelings of ambiguity and the range of emotions that can accompany change. Consider the losses that Nerida has experienced. Apart from the obvious loss of health, she has also lost a sense of trust in her body. She has missed out on so much of what her peers take for granted. She feels alienated, isolated, fearful, and outside the mainstream.

A broad understanding of loss as the trigger for grief is of great importance for nurses. Not only does it alert us to what may be a covert element in the suffering of those in our care; it also provides perspectives for becoming more acutely aware of the impact of loss in life and our own attitudes, thoughts, feelings, and behavioural responses in our personal encounters with loss and grief, death and dying.

Among the most difficult tasks we are all likely to face in life is handling loss—our own personal losses and helping those people we care for who suffer losses. The difficulty lies not only in attending to the upheaval and practicalities occasioned by the loss event but also in managing the emotional pain precipitated by the loss. Difficulties are further compounded when, for instance, the loss is related to a slowly manifesting condition that often involves adjustment to a different body image, or to the loss of hopes and dreams due to, say, infertility, relationship breakdown, or miscarriage; that is, when the loss is non-finite.

# Non-finite loss

Pause for a moment to contemplate the loss and grief associated with the following sample of scenarios found in the literature. They may be situations with which you identify on a personal level—loss of a limb (Kenny & Schultz 1993); stillbirth (Lewis & Page 1978); relinquishment of a child through adoption (Condon 1986, Winkler & van Keppel 1984); or elective abortion (Peppers & Knapp 1980). Perhaps, like Nerida, you have had your life complicated by a chronic illness from childhood. Possibly you are acquainted with losses that parallel the process of human growth and development (Schneider 1984, Sullender 1985), or the loss of shared paths, dreams, and wishes that are an integral part of development, as Carol Shields described (1997, p 131):

> To get better. To live. To grow up. To be like everyone else. Isn't that what we all want in the end?

These are but a few examples of what we have defined as non-finite loss. We coined the term non-finite loss to refer to those losses for which there is no clearly marked conclusion; so that the extent of loss becomes more apparent with the passage of time, shattering our hopes and wishes for the future, our ideals and expectations.

There is a strong theoretical basis for our conceptualisation of non-finite loss in the literature (Berger & Luckmann 1966, Bowlby 1980, Freud 1917, Horowitz 1983, 1988, 1990, Marris 1986, Olshansky 1962, Parkes 1972, 1986, Rochlin 1965). Non-finite loss is an umbrella term for many situations in life, affecting young and old alike. Who then might experience non-finite loss? The answer is anyone who experiences the irrevocable loss of that which plays a central role in who they perceive themselves to be. Recurrent grief throughout life about a loss—be it a person, wish, goal, health—identifies the loss as non-finite.

Nerida's loss is non-finite in nature—it is enduring and evolutionary. Her diabetes is incurable. During her life, its meaning and significance has slowly evolved. The part that her illness has played and will play in her life is revealed only over time, with each stage of cognitive and socioemotional development adding breadth to the meaning of this condition. She needs to be allowed to reflect on the non-finite nature of her loss, the trauma it had involved for a 5-year-old, and how she is going to blend it into her present world and be able to communicate her situation to the people she meets. Given appropriate support, this is achievable. Family, friends, and professionals face the challenge of helping her give words to all the isolation and fears that she has been harbouring. Nerida's parents have also experienced non-finite loss.

## Case study . . . *continued*

When Nerida was diagnosed with diabetes, her parents were shocked and distressed. They were both well educated, but unfamiliar with how to communicate this illness to their daughter. Unfortunately, they were too up-front: 'She must be told what she has.' They were unable to understand the cognitive limitations of a 5-year-old. They were frightened of what might happen if Nerida did not follow her regimen. They pushed the same line inadvertently, or sometimes as a threat. They were constantly on tenterhooks. They expected her to take responsibility for her injections early—too early for a young child still scared of body integrity issues. Her parents took it for granted that she would get used to it. They did not understand that Nerida's adaptation was hindered by her fears, rather than by her own relationship with the condition of diabetes or mastery of it. As Nerida developed, she kept her private world of diabetes secret. She did not join any groups that might allow her to talk about her fears or to feel normal. Only one or two friends knew, and those times when she brought it up with her parents, their anxious expressions cut off any further opening up. How could they understand diabetes, her world? They did not have diabetes. Their response was repetitive: it could have been so much worse.

Nerida's parents could not feel her grief, because they had never dealt with their own grief. Through adolescence, she often acted out against this repressed fear of her diabetes. Her anxiety about it took over. And there were other repercussions. While in Nerida's mind her parents never forgot about it, her sister, Shirley, was jealous of it. Anxious enquiry would follow any of Nerida's off-days, while Shirley would roll her eyes as though Nerida was basking in the attention. Shirley often felt short-changed, because her sister's condition meant that she had lost out on a lot, too. She loved Nerida, but hated being part of a household that was so different to that of her peers. It made it very hard for her to make friends and her parents always seemed to be fretting over Nerida and her future. She felt isolated and unimportant sometimes.

Nerida's loss, and that of her family, is a loss across the lifespan. To summarise, loss that spans a lifetime can be thought of in two different ways: losses that are an inevitable part of living, including the dying trajectory, and those that are characterised by a cycle of chronicity, as in Nerida's case. Loss and grief are inexorably linked, but when there is a ceaseless interplay between *what was* or *what might have been* and *what is*, the grieving is likely to become complicated. One consequence of this is that people like Nerida may have no recourse but to avoid their grief. This avoidance may allow them to salvage hopes for the future—a type of adaptation. It is of concern, however, that in this safety net of avoidance, the actual intensity of the emotions attached to diagnosis at any age may be missed or overlooked by family members and professional caregivers.

The provision of psychological support services in cases of irrevocable loss is particularly complicated. Individuals are likely to put their grief on hold, particularly in social settings. Recognising the process of adaptation behind an individual's defences is a challenge. In cases where there is no doubt that there has been a psychological trauma, nurses may seek guidance and debriefing so that they can assist these individuals.

# The impact of loss

When we think in terms of the whole person, with needs and reactions at the physical, psychological, social, emotional, and spiritual levels, it becomes clear that the impact of our losses can have a profound effect on a person's life. The extent of that impact is a very individual matter. It is influenced by a large range of factors, including the nature of the loss and whether it was expected, anticipated, or sudden. Psychological factors influencing the impact of loss include personality, developmental stage in life, outlook on life, how previous losses were managed, assumptions about life that are challenged by the loss, ability to find meaning, and capacity or readiness to adapt to the change. Peoples' experience of grief could also be influenced by their family, cultural and religious backgrounds.

Early experiences of attachment provide us with a very important blueprint, not only in terms of our fundamental response to loss but also our ability to trust other people. This trust applies to the care that others offer and to a general belief that there are many good and caring people around. According to Bowlby (1988), healthy positive attachments that can largely be taken for granted in infancy develop a secure psychological base in an individual. This secure base provides a necessary emotional harbour to enable children to develop their skills to handle the inevitable losses, frustrations, and complex human emotions inherent in daily life.

Thus, early attachment experiences generate innate assumptions about the world as it should be, both now and in the future. When those assumptions are threatened by loss events, learned coping mechanisms are activated. For those individuals lacking a secure base to cling to, the outcome can be overwhelming. It may be useful to briefly reflect on what Nerida's experience with her family has generated in terms of her assumptions about receiving or asking for care. Given that Nerida's parents have assigned a level of responsibility to their daughter for the management of her illness, we can generate a number of hypotheses about what Nerida has come to expect from other caregivers and from herself. She has been expected to be 'tough', she has adopted an exterior that camouflages her insecurities, and she does not trust that expressing her fears is reasonable (that is, she fears being judged negatively). Nerida's story highlights the significant role of parents and professionals in helping individuals deal with their illness and the losses surrounding it. Personal experiences lead those who are ill to a framework within which they interpret their experience of loss, hopes and dreams, expectations about how the world should be, and deeply entrenched fears and attitudes about events they have learnt to dread (Bruce & Schultz 2001, 2003). These fears and discrepancies combine to produce a dynamic that can, in turn, pose a grave threat to our sense of identity, particularly when a severe loss is suffered.

# Loss and family

It is important to consider how loss influences a family (Bronfenbrenner 1979, Hartman 1978). In each family there are alliances, patterns of interacting, different ways of handling pressures and stresses. Losses occur to whole families and to individual family members at various stages of the family's life. The nature of the relationships within the family, whether characterised by closeness, alienation, or dependency are factors to be taken into account by those whose role it is to support each family member in their care. The role and function of individual members within the family system and within the overall societal environment also plays a part as people wrestle with their loss.

A loss in the family may be to do with a degenerative disease, permanent injury, congenital malformation, or loss through death, to give but a few examples where every member suffers and is likely to be affected by the trauma. It introduces change in the family dynamics, with a loss of normal patterns. For example, an adult son or daughter may assume the primary caring role previously held by their mother or father, or a sibling like Shirley may feel uncared for as the focus of attention is necessarily given to another family member. For further examples of the impact of loss on individuals and families, see *The Caregiving Years* by Schultz & Schultz (1998).

There are differing gender realities that can be traced to differing sets of circumstances, background experiences, and formative processes. Chapter 4 considered how gender can influence health and illness experiences, and it is also clear that gender can profoundly influence responses to loss. For instance, some individuals, noticeably males (Golden 1996), seem to translate aspects of a personal tragedy into a doing role. Often, while a mother struggles with the intensity of what she faces due to a chronic condition her child endures, the father responds with an action plan external to the household. It is as if some males seek to find ways out of the intensity of the family trauma and the woman cannot imagine any escape (Bruce & Schultz 2002).

## Nurses and loss

Apart from acquiring a theoretical framework to assist in considering issues of loss and grief, it is essential for effective and professional nurses to be prepared to examine their own personal experience of loss and to gain insight into their own grief reactions. This will help them to understand the grief process and its impact on others. Gilliland & James (1988) considered these steps to be prerequisites for crisis workers and caregivers. These authors also listed effective communication skills, commitment to supporting the grieving person (and family where appropriate), and possession of knowledge of one's personal limits as essential attributes. Your unique personal pattern of how, or how not to, show pain and feelings is of particular significance as these patterns exert enormous influence on the capacity to express grief (Bruce & Schultz 2001, 2004).

Nurses need to reflect on their willingness to be available for the experience of grieving in another individual. The capacity to be with or endure another individual's strong emotions relies on a nurse's willingness to endure grief and the expression of strong emotions, while also respecting the place of, and expression of, sad feelings and enormous tracts of disappointment as a normal part of loss. To this end, you are invited to reflect on personal issues of your own, as you study the sections on loss and grief. Try to pinpoint times when you have been confronted with the strong emotions of another person. Try to recapture and picture a sense of the physical feelings inside your body—and search for the words you usually find yourself drawing upon.

# Loss and grief in life

This section considers loss and grief as part of human existence. The nature of griefwork is described, common myths about grieving are explored and the manifestations of grief are discussed.

## Griefwork

Grief is the universally recognised response to loss. This process is often so intense that it has been referred to in the literature as griefwork. Bowlby (1980) described this work as the redefinition of self and situation. The occurrence of a traumatic event in our lives threatens our reality; we are forced to change our perception of the world we have grown attached to—the world as it should be, and to engage in a painful, and frequently prolonged, redefinition of the reality that we took for granted. For Nerida, since she was a young child, diabetes has been slowly demonstrating how her life differs from her peers and how it may encumber her future. She is forced to modify her expectations of her self and what the world can offer her, bit by bit.

This redefinition means facing up to reality; it means giving up old versions of self, while re-establishing identity: 'Who am I without the lost object or person?' There is a search for meaning, trying to make sense of the new world and why it has happened. This is particularly so when individuals are seeking a reason for why they have been personally afflicted.

There is no doubt that grieving is a complex process. Not so widely recognised, however, is the grief of persons for whom non-finite loss is a constant presence, or surfaces in a diminished sense of identity, brought about by childhood or adolescent setbacks or by chronic illness. We have likened the experience of non-finite loss to living permanently in a house haunted by a ghost. The house represents the world as it is emerging after the loss event (less than the ideal) and the ghost is the world that once had been expected and planned upon (the ideal world).

Individuals like Nerida who are grieving the non-finite loss associated with chronic illness are grappling with relinquishing ideals or certain ways of being in the world which are normally taken for granted. The obstinate hovering ghost may be that of a normal child, the healthy fit and able body— the lifestyle which may have surrounded a child who would eventually become independent and cease relying on the parent's proximity. *Nerida and her parents are classic examples of people living in such a haunted house. As for all persons living with chronic conditions, they are experiencing non-finite loss.*

## Myths about grieving

By far the most popular and well-known explanation of the grieving process is that of Elisabeth Kübler Ross (1969). Despite many authors pointing to more complex contexts of loss, the work of Kübler Ross (1969) has received greater attention, possibly because of its more accessible approach to grieving and to its direct link to the subject of death and dying. She applied stage theory, popularised by Freud (1917) and Piaget (1951), to the process of grieving. Because of the widespread attention to her work, the processes of grief and loss and death and dying were more openly discussed (Kastenbaum 1982, p 111). Her contribution did much to eventually break down the previous taboos related to openly discussing such topics. For instance, writing in 1985, Kalish described the lengths to which people would go to avoid discussing death or talking openly with a dying person. Closer to home, an Australian survey by Burney-Banfield (1994) found that death education was not widely included in nursing curricula. Fortunately, there has been a major shift, leading to a far greater acknowledgment at many levels (for example, McGrath et al 1999).

Kübler Ross based her insights on her clinical experiences as a psychiatrist working with dying patients, describing the grieving process in terms of denial, anger, bargaining, depression, and acceptance. Despite the cautions expressed in analyses such as Kastenbaum's (1982), the stage approach retains popular appeal: it provides structure and insight into the dying process, thereby reducing anxiety and providing a sense of security, both for the grieving person and for the professional helper. However, there are serious problems with the stage perspective on grief, in that it invites an interpretation of an uninterrupted linear progression between one stage and the next, and a disregard for individual differences. However we would argue that far from linear, the grieving process may well be cyclical, and having no fixed pattern.

Whatever the loss situation, there is a real danger that in using stage-based theories of loss, there will be a stereotyping of a person's grieving response, and of interpreting verbal and non-verbal behaviours in such a way as to make them fit neatly into stages or 'boxes'. In the process of doing that, it is likely that nurses may miss out on understanding a given situation more closely or place inappropriate expectations upon their patients and family members.

Our preferred term is adaptation—which is an entirely achievable and possible goal, whereas emotional acceptance may not ever be realised. This is actually what Nerida is grappling with: trying to emotionally accept her chronic illness in her life that she instinctively wants to rage against and reject. According to Nerida, she feels robbed! Our prime thought regarding the use of the notion of 'acceptance' as a goal of grieving is that it may well be impossible.

## Manifestations of grief

Although the individuality of responses to loss vary, there are commonalities to be found in griefwork. You may recognise feelings you yourself have perhaps experienced—sadness, anger, guilt, anxiety, loneliness, yearning, helplessness, shock, even relief. These are some of the reactions Worden (2002, pp 7–24) listed as normal manifestations of grief, along with physical sensations (for example, lack of energy and tightness in the throat), cognitions (for example, disbelief, confusion, distractedness), and behaviours (for example, sleep and appetite disturbance, crying, social withdrawal, or overactivity).

What might be considered as abnormal grief? Drawing distinctions between abnormal and normal is difficult. In a straightforward grieving process, the manifestations of grief wax and wane but generally, over time, there is a movement towards adaptation to the evolving new reality. In more complicated grief reactions, this general abating of strong difficult emotions may not occur. There may be obstacles to adaptation, due to the lack of inner coping resources in the grieving individuals. It is in these instances that professional support may be necessary.

In our research and practice, we have observed ever-evolving cycles and recurring states of mind for those individuals who are grieving non-finite loss. Apart from the complications associated with the attempts of some persons to avoid their grief or to deny themselves any entitlement to grieve, we have identified five reactivating themes characterised as follows:

- shock and detachment from reality: 'This can't be happening';
- protest: 'There must be a way out of this mess';
- defiance: 'I can fix this';
- despair: 'I cannot fix this'; and
- integration: 'I have no choice but to make the best of this'.

Interestingly, we have observed that shock as a theme can be reactivated in varying forms and degrees of intensity, despite the time elapsed. For instance, a rediagnosis of any disease, be it a complication or a further tumour, is sufficient to reactivate this cycle. If the person has sustained a considerable period of time without evidence of the condition and has started to entertain ideas of invincibility, there will be shock.

Integration is a term worth examining. What does it mean? What is the best possible emotional scenario or outcome? Let's draw on the example of Nerida. As a young adult, and in the pursuit of being connected with her friends, she pushes the limits of her condition. Inevitably, she learns that this defiance has a high price—a week in hospital follows. Over time, she will integrate this learning, with the condition becoming part of her decision about what things she can do. Of course, this is terribly simplistic—the emotional pain will be arduous.

We would urge readers to be sceptical about the degree of integration that can be achieved. It is difficult to imagine individuals with a chronic condition blandly integrating a future that involves continuing pain or frightening traumatic images involving themselves or a loved one. It would appear to be adaptive to employ an emotional shield (Snyder 1989). For instance, as therapists, we have observed that hope hovers in the background, while the yearning for 'what might have been' persists as the benchmark against which loss is experienced. It is amid this conflict that individuals often do reach what best could be described as an adaptive relationship with their loss (Bruce & Schultz 2001, p 163). Nerida eventually reached that point, but that is not to say that she did not frequently, and often painfully, revisit every one of those characteristic themes mentioned earlier.

## Determinants of the length and intensity of grief

There are no rules about how a person should grieve. However, there are factors unique to each person that influence the grieving process. Some of these have been listed under the impact of loss, but a further helpful way of thinking about this issue of individuality was proposed by Parkes (1972). He suggested that our past, our present, and our future all contribute to a person's particular response to loss.

Parkes (1972) proposed that current factors influencing a person's response to loss include financial status, support systems, and level of resilience. The next chapter explores the concept of resilience in some depth, defining it as a person's capacity to deal with adversity. Subsequent to a loss experience, factors that are likely to influence the length and intensity of our grief include the social support available (or not), secondary stressors and, importantly, emergent life opportunities; that is, opportunities for emotional relief. Support is an important element and an aspect within which nurses have a key role to play.

As we've previously noted, there is no guarantee that resolution of grief will occur. For some it may; for others, the best that might be hoped for is an outcome of adaptation. Adaptation is often an ongoing task, when an individual realises that he or she can manage his or her world, that is, the real world, not the one that should have been (Bruce & Schultz 2001).

The road towards adaptation is facilitated by nurses, and other caring professionals, who demonstrate a capacity to understand the intensity of the emotions and the rights of their patients to feel what they feel. It is important not to exert any extraneous pressure through premature and unreasonable talks of acceptance. Well informed family and friends often assist in this process but, as Nerida's parents illustrated, good intentions are not always enough.

## Support on the journey of grief

One of the greatest challenges confronting nurses is to be able to support their clients or patients as they face living with their grief. The extent of the challenge increases when we remember that, instinctively, grief is contagious and frightens others (Axelsson 2002, p 296).

The ability to provide support for the grieving person requires:

- courage and dedication;
- an appreciation of what is meant by loss across the lifespan, for individuals and their family;
- an understanding of the dynamics underlying grief;
- the cultivation in ourselves and others of effective strategies to adapt to loss and grief;
- effective communication skills: listening, responding appropriately, verbal and non-verbal validation, as well as qualities of being such as touch, humour, expressive art, and reciprocity;

- referral skills and knowing one's own limits; and
- taking care of your own needs and ensuring access to a support person or group for yourself.

This chapter has provided you with knowledge about loss and grief based on relevant literature. Your own experience, attitudes, and self-awareness add breadth to that knowledge, as does your specialised training and technical skills. Brammer and Macdonald (1996) talked about how a helper's personality combines with specific skills to produce a powerful formula for effective caregiving. As a nurse, you have the privilege of applying such a profound force to support those in your care who are grieving. Effective interpersonal skills in relating are essential and a few examples of particular relevance to situations of loss and grief are briefly discussed below.

# Reflective listening and the validation of your client's emotions

These are helpful ways of reducing the intensity of feelings otherwise amplified if they remain held inside. In chronic conditions that create situations of non-finite loss, you will have the onerous task of reassuring these individuals of their entitlement to feel grief and to feel the range of feelings that we have described. You will be their source of validation. Encourage them to avoid self-recriminations about feeling ongoing anxiety and grief.

Given the emotional intensity that often surrounds traumatic loss, even carefully chosen words can wreak havoc. You will have become relatively desensitised to the words describing procedures. Use careful language to marginalise the negative consequences and, importantly, continue to check your language, your anxiety levels, and what is being conveyed to patients.

In those times when you must respect silence—make sure your body language and facial expressions continue to offer validation.

To conclude, we refer to Gabrielle Bortoluzzi's account of facing death (1994), in which ten strategies were listed by which personal and professional relationships can be enriched. The following points from her work provide a useful summary of what has been covered in this chapter, and some clear guidelines for nurses working with those who are confronting their own death or the death of someone they love (pp 8–9):

- Communicate sensitively without clichéd comment.
- Respect the individual's unique feelings and the timing of their expression.
- Avoid indulging in 'fix it' mode.
- Understand the theory of the grieving process, but never impose it on the individual in your care.
- Value the life and contribution of the person in the present time.
- Respect and support each individual's coping style.
- Communicate confidence in therapeutic skills.

- Understand the literature on loss and grief and understand your own feelings about death and dying.
- Acknowledge the importance of the loss to the sufferer; avoid comparison with the loss of other patients.
- A blend of honesty and versions of reality that offer relief or hope are vital parts of any communication.

## Tutorial questions

1. What losses have you personally experienced?
2. Do you think talking about death will make you more or less at ease about your own or others' death?
3. What do you consider to be the main prerequisites for supporting those who are grieving?
4. What do the following terms mean to you:
   a) lifespan loss;
   b) griefwork; and
   c) nonfinite loss.
5. The loss of function of a member of a family means that grief is part of that family's experience, both collectively and as individuals. Discuss this statement.
6. What would you like to say to Nerida? Her sister? Her parents?

*Acknowledgment.* We are grateful to our colleague, Chris Hall, Director, Centre for Grief Education, Monash Medical Centre, Victoria, for his assistance in searching for recent Australian literature relevant to our topic.

## References

Axelsson M 2002 *April Witch*. L Schenck (Translation), Hodden, Sydney (Original work published 1997)

Berger PL, Luckmann T 1966 *The Social Construction of Reality*. Penguin Press, London

Bortoluzzi G 1994 Facing death: A personal perspective. *NZ Journal of Physiotherapy* April:6–9

Bowlby J 1980 *Loss, sadness and depression*. Penguin Press, London

Bowlby J 1988 *A secure base: Clinical applications of attachment theory*. Routledge, London

Brammer LM, Macdonald G 1996 *The helping relationship: Process and skills*, 6th edn. Allyn and Bacon, Boston, MA

Bronfenbrenner U 1979 *The ecology of human development*. Harvard University Press, Cambridge, M

Bruce EJ, Schultz CL 2001 *Nonfinite loss and grief: A psychoeducational approach*. Maclennan Petty, Sydney

Bruce EJ, Schultz CL 2002 Non-finite loss and challenges to communication between parents and professionals. *British Journal of Special Education* 29(1):9–13

Bruce EJ, Schultz CL 2003 Block and Tackle ™ Groupwork: Psychological techniques for working with nonfinite and traumatic loss in family settings. (Available from Authors)

Bruce EJ, Schultz CL  2004 *Through loss*. ACER, Melbourne

Burney-Banfield S 1994 Preparing students for their patient's deaths. *Australian Journal of Advanced Nursing* 11:24–28

Condon JT 1986 Psychological disability in women who relinquish a baby for adoption. *The Medical Journal of Australia* 144:117–119

Freud S 1917 Mourning and melancholia, in *Sigmund Freud: Collected papers, vol 4*. Basic Books, New York

Gilliland BE, James RK 1988 *Crisis intervention strategies*. Brooks/Cole, Pacific Grove, CA

Golden T 1996 *Swallowed by a snake*. Golden Healing Publishing, Maryland, USA

Hartman A 1978 Diagrammatic assessment of family relationships. *Social Casework* 59:469–476

Horowitz MJ 1983 Psychological responses to serious life events. In: S Breznitz (ed), *The Denial of Stress*. International Universities Press, Madison, CT, pp 129–159

Horowitz MJ 1988 *Introduction to psychodynamics: A new synthesis*. Basic Books, New York

Horowitz MJ 1990 A model of mourning: Change in schemas of self and other. *Journal of the American Psychoanalytic Association* 38:297–324

Janicki MP, Dalton AJ (eds) 1999 *Aging, Dementia, and Intellectual Disabilities: A Handbook*. Taylor & Francis, Philadelphia

Kalish RA 1985 *Death, grief, and caring relationships*, 2nd edn. Brooke/Cole, Monetrey, CA

Kastenbaum R 1982 Do we die in stages? In: Wilcox SG, Sutton M (eds), *Understanding death and dying: An interdisciplinary approach*. 2nd edn. pp 109–117. Mayfield, Palo Alto, CA

Kenny PB, Schultz CL 1993 The grief reaction of an individual to amputation. *Australian Orthotic Prosthetic Magazine* 8(2):19–21

Kübler Ross E 1969 *On death and dying*. Macmillan, New York

Lewis E, Page A 1978 Failure to mourn a stillbirth: An overlooked catastrophe. *British Journal of Medical Psychology* 51:237–241

Marris P 1986 *Loss and change*, 2nd edn. Routledge & Kegan-Paul, London

McGrath P, Yates P, Clinton M, Hart G 1999 What should I say? Qualitative findings on dilemmas in palliative care nursing. *The Hospice Journal* 14(2)17–33

O'Connor J, Jeavons S 2003 Nurses' perceptions of critical incidents. *Journal of Advanced Nursing* 41(1):53–62

Olshansky S 1962 Chronic sorrow: A response to having a mentally defective child. *Social Casework* 43:190–193

Parkes CM 1972 Components of the reaction to loss of a limb, spouse, or home. *Journal of Psychosomatic Research* 16:343–349

Parkes CM 1986 What becomes of redundant world models. A contribution to the study of adaptation to change. *British Journal of Medical Psychology* 48:131–137

Peppers LG, Knapp RJ 1980 *Motherhood and mourning perinatal death*. Praegar Publishers, New York

Piaget J 1951 *The child's conception of the world*. Littlefield Adams, Savage, MD (Original work published 1929)

Rochlin G 1965 *Grief and discontents: The forces of change*. Churchill, London JA

**141**

# Living with Illness

Schneider J 1984 *Stress, loss, and grief.* University Park Press, Baltimore

Schultz CL, Schultz NC 1998 *The caregiving years.* ACER, Melbourne, Victoria

Shakespeare W 1943 Macbeth. In: WJ Craig (ed), *The complete works of William Shakespeare*, Rev edn. Oxford University Press, London

Shields C 1997 *Larry's Party.* Fourth Estate, London

Snyder CR 1989 Reality negotiation. From excuses to hope and beyond. *Journal of Social and Clinical Psychology* 8(2):130–157

Sullender RC 1985 *Grief and growth: Pastoral resources for emotional and spiritual growth.* Paulist Press, New Jersey

Winkler R, van Keppel M 1984 Relinquishing mothers in adoption. *Australian Institute of Family Studies*, Melbourne, Victoria

Worden W 2002 *Grief counseling and grief therapy*, 3rd edn. Springer, New York

# Chapter 11

## Journeys through Illness: Suffering and Resilience

*Kristine Martin-McDonald and Cath Rogers-Clark*

**This chapter:**

- explores the notion of living with chronic illness as a journey;
- explores the concepts of enduring and uncertainty as aspects of the suffering associated with living with chronic illness;
- defines resilience;
- explores the ways in which people develop and use resilient strategies in the face of chronic illness;
- describes survivorship as an outcome of resilience; and
- discusses the role of nurses and other caring professionals in relation to supporting a person through their suffering, and to develop their resilience in the face of that suffering.

This chapter is focused on illness experiences. Illness experiences are inevitably challenging for the person with the illness, and may involve periods of often quite intense suffering. At the same time, there is ample evidence that many people living with illness, especially chronic illness, learn to manage both their illness and their own responses to it. Suffering and resilience, then, are major dimensions of the illness journey. Both are discussed in this chapter. As was noted in Chapter 8, there is a variety of publications written by people with chronic illness, in which their own experiences are detailed. Nurses have much to learn from these publications as well as from those who talk to us about their illness journeys. If we will only listen, we will hear how they have suffered, but also how they survive each day and get on with their lives as well as they can in the shadow of illness.

The analogy that living with an illness is like being on a journey helps to explain the diversity of illness experiences. Illness journeys can be short or long, but are more than likely to involve periods of suffering, which may take any number of forms, as well as times when things seem to be easier and the person with an illness feels positive and is coping well. There is no one pathway through illness, and people live with their diseases in different ways. Some will find that their journey is direct and swift, whilst others experience detours, delays, and obstacles. Some with be completely cured of their disease, others will live with chronic illness for the rest of their lives, and some will not survive.

However the traveller proceeds, any journey through illness can expose a person to the unexpected, moving a person into the unknown and the uncertain, almost like being in an eclipse. This is a place where suffering is intensified and any view of the journey's destination becomes shrouded. An eclipse places one in that moment alone, which is like no other moment. The traveller is likely to have little control at this time. For some, the journey is stalled in the eclipse, and marked by continuing and sometimes unbearable suffering. For others, the eclipse ends as the person develops their resilience and becomes a survivor.

As in all journeys, roads may loop back on themselves, returning the traveller to the point of eclipse, at times when the challenges are simply too difficult. Ultimately, however, the traveller requires personal energy derived from within and outside of them in order to maintain a focus on their destination, wherever that may be.

This chapter will explore the concepts of suffering, resilience and survivorship in relation to the story of a man living on renal dialysis. The chapter will also consider the roles of the nurse and other caring professionals in supporting and encouraging the person living with illness through their journey.

## Case study: Gary's story

I was 32 years old when I was told that I had kidney disease and I would need dialysis one day. When I was 46 I suddenly lost weight, felt tired, my eyes were black, I felt haggard and was pale. I lost so much weight. I thought 'Struth! What is wrong?' I thought it was sinister like cancer. I went to see the renal specialist and I was told to start dialysis.

I was infuriated. The specialist arranged for me to visit a renal unit a week later. I saw people hooked up to machines. I thought 'Oh, God! this is not for me.' I spoke to people about dialysis. It was terrifying to look at. 'Oh no, not me, God.' I was shocked, confused. It looked overpowering. 'From now on, life is stuffed. Being tied to a machine. Life is going to be hell' is what I thought. In the back of my mind, it seemed like going to boarding school to me, locked up for years. I was angry. Couldn't put up with anybody. Bad, short-tempered. It was terrible.

I felt like dying. My skin was all yellow. I looked terrible. The doctors and nurses wanted me on dialysis as soon as possible. I'd say, 'No, I'm not ready yet.' I wouldn't be in it. I kept putting dialysis off and putting it off.

I was much sicker than I thought. Finally, it just got too much for me. When it hit me, it was like hitting a brick wall. I just got too sick. I was very ugly on the world.

They told me I would be better within 2 months of dialysis. But 2 weeks, that's all it took. I noticed it straight away. I'm stupid, stupid. It was ridiculous putting it off for so long.

I was a bit apprehensive. I hated needles. I thought 'Oh well, I have to cop it.' The nurses knew what they were doing. Accepting that I needed dialysis was the hardest part.

The only thing that I worry about is potassium, because if I have too much it will kill me. Not having chocolate and things like that aren't a problem because I don't like the stuff anyway but I had to give up cola drinks because it brings up your potassium. I love my beer, but I don't booze much now. I don't want to overdo how much fluid I take.

A good day is when I'm active and I don't think about dialysis. Bad days are when I feel terribly drowsy, off-colour and heavy in the head. I have to take things more slowly. I am a bit cranky. The more time I have to think about dialysis the worse I get on bad days.

I've learnt to take each day as it comes. I'm pretty sure that I'll get a kidney transplant one day but I know it's going to take time. Sometimes I still think 'why me?', but other times I think 'why not me?'. Compared to a lot of other people, I'm pretty well. It could have got a lot worse and I'm better off than many.

# Enduring, uncertainly and suffering

This section discusses enduring, uncertainty and suffering as key features of the experience of illness.

## Enduring

When an illness occurs, the impact on a person's life may be so intense that dealing with it is beyond the capacity of their normal coping responses. It may feel like being thrown into the unknown. A coping response to this stage of the journey has been labelled as *enduring* (Morse 1997). Enduring is defined as the way a person gets through this immediate reaction to the situation. It is innate, rather than learned, with a focus on 'hanging on' and protecting oneself. It is focused on the here-and-now, not the future and it involves a temporary void of emotions. Like numbness, emotionally and intellectually the situation remains temporarily incomprehensible.

A normal human response during and beyond a life-changing crisis, such as an illness, is to attempt to understand what has happened and why it has occurred. When the level of knowing about the illness is limited to awareness without full comprehension, the person enters the stage of *enduring*.

For as long as he could, Gary delayed the commencement of dialysis despite the deterioration of his health. His fear of losing control to the dialysis process and the health professionals motivated him to delay dialysis until he was simply too unwell. On commencement of dialysis, Gary moved to *enduring* as a way of coping with, and accepting his dependence on the health professionals:

> I tried to shut my eyes and pretend it would all be over soon. It was
> awful, but I just had to hang in there otherwise I'd be a goner.

At this stage, people may be concerned about 'losing it' through embarrassing or unacceptable behaviours. They may try to 'put on a brave face',
to avoid behaviours such as uncontrollable crying, rage in the form of
profanities, shouting, or even physical acts of aggression. This is important,
because 'losing it' in such ways often brings about some kind of institutional
sanctions against the offender (Dewar & Morse 1995). For example, people
may be labelled as 'problem patients', or 'attention seekers'.

To move through this stage of *enduring*, strategies may be employed as an
attempt to regain a sense of control over their lives. For example, the person
may direct their energies to something that takes their mind off what is
happening to them. Whilst on dialysis, Gary shared his concerns about how his
wife would manage the business whilst he was away. This seemed to occupy a
lot of his attention. He felt the need to retain significant involvement:

> When I'm in the renal unit, I'm either joking with the nurses or using
> that time to make phone orders for the stock we need in the shop.

At this point of the journey, so much is unknown. For example, suddenly
a person may feel that their body is a stranger to them, and can no longer
be trusted. They may no longer be certain of the limits of their body's
endurance, or their emotional capacity to handle these challenges positively.
This means people who are *enduring* are living in uncertain territory that
threatens to overwhelm them. Gary lacked the required knowledge to
manage his dialysis regime. In fact, the amount that he did not know and
understand was daunting to him:

> You are nervous because it's all so new and you're super careful.
> Probably too careful, 'cause you don't want to forget anything and
> you don't want to make a mistake. It (dialysis) seems to try and
> overwhelm you.

## Uncertainty

Over time the reality of the illness situation, and the inevitable changes that
accompany this, sink in and the person moves into a stage known as
*uncertainty*. Uncertainty is that stage of the journey where a person's past life
is lost but the person is unsure of what is to come, and how they will respond
to whatever challenges arise. For example, related to employment, people
with an illness may lose their capacity to work, either because employers
may not tolerate time out needed for treatment such as dialysis, and/or
because of reduced physical or mental capacity:

> Struth, I've got so much to learn. How the heck am I ever going to
> be able to deal with all of this. Not only do I lose three days a week
> to dialysis, but I can't drink with me mates anymore because of fluid

restrictions and I have to make damned sure I don't get infections in my fistula, so I can't play footy anymore. It's just not bloody fair.

During this stage, a sense of personal control may seem to ebb away. Tentative goals are often unattainable, simply because the person does not know how to achieve them because of the current state of their illness. For example, plans for a holiday may be awry when an unanticipated complication occurs just days before the departure date:

I love travelling. Done heaps as a young bloke. I've been waiting for my kids to get old enough before doing anymore. My plans are stuffed now because I have to be in the dialysis unit three days a week. The nurses say I can have holidays at other towns with renal units, but they're booked out months in advance. It's just too much bother to have to organise it because who knows what condition I'll be in then.

When a person's sense of control is completely lost, and the losses a person has endured feel too great, the illness journey is likely to move into the stage of suffering.

## Suffering

There is an overwhelming emotional experience when a person is engulfed by the magnitude of what is happening and they are plunged fully into *suffering*. It is an experience of the total self, a personal, subjective experience that may vary from simple, transitory discomfort to extreme angst and distress. The 'threat' of suffering relates to the disintegration of the 'self' as known to the person and commences when a person becomes aware that their future will be different to the path they had chosen or envisaged. Thus, suffering does not necessarily commence at the time that function worsens for someone who has a chronic illness, but rather when they become aware of what the future holds or fails to hold for them.

The attributes of suffering convey it as an individualised, subjective and complex experience when a person loses or is at risk of losing control over his/her situation or life. The meaning that suffering brings to a person's life is intensely negative in nature where integrity, autonomy and personal identity are lost or under threat. Sufferers' coping mechanisms are taxed beyond their effectiveness.

Suffering is one of the most profound and disturbing human experiences. And yet, the term 'suffering' is trivialised by its frequent misuse. For example, this term is often incorrectly used by laypeople, marketers and even some health disciplines to mean 'diagnosed with', such as 'suffering from hayfever', or 'suffering from influenza'. Such use of the term usually focuses on observable and measurable pathophysiology and has a tendency to overlook all the aspects of a person that are affected by an illness, such as the cognitive, social, affective and spiritual consequences of that illness.

Equally misleading is the use of terms such as 'anxiety', 'stress', 'distress' and 'depression' synonymously with suffering. These descriptors fail to capture the potency and intensity of the experience of suffering. Additionally, using these terms suggests that the distress is somehow unhealthy and unnatural, and should be diagnosed and treated as a mental illness rather than a normal human response to an overwhelming situation:

> Everything I wanted to do is gone. From now on, life is stuffed. Being tied to a machine. Life is going to be hell.

A person who is suffering may seek to find some meaning in it, to answer the question 'why me?'. In the quest to find an answer to that question, a sufferer's values, beliefs and identity are challenged and altered, as they are no longer the person they thought they were. The experience of suffering may be related to different aspects of an illness, such as: sickness and treatment, for example, pain; care provision, for example, being deprived of power or dignity, or adequate pain relief; and to each person's unique life and existence, for example, the tension between feelings of hope and hopelessness. The different levels of suffering can be heard in Gary's comments below.

Suffering related to the sickness:

> I felt like dying. My skin was all yellow. I looked terrible.

> I don't feel like a normal person. I just haven't got the energy.

Suffering related to the provision of care:

> The doctors and nurses wanted me on dialysis as soon as possible.

> The doctors and nurses are the experts and I don't want to learn too much otherwise I might want to tell them what to do.

Suffering related to a person's situation:

> When you have something like this, it affects every facet of your life . . . It's just everything. It's like a snowball thing. It just gets bigger and bigger . . . I still think 'why me?'. I have my ups and downs. Like, what could be, where I could be, where I could be working.

Suffering shapes our family and friend networks and how we can live in the world (Kleinman 1991). There is a sense of not being connected to others because suffering isolates and, at times, even alienates the sufferers from the community. Thus social relationships are altered and, at times, family and friends become inattentive, or withdraw completely. This exacerbates the loss and suffering and social isolation experienced:

> A lot of our friends have just deserted us . . . I feel alienated. I mean a five minute phone call once every month. How much does that take? And they don't even do that. There's no excuse. It's them I guess, not being able to cope with the way I am. I mean, I haven't changed. I'm still the same person, it's just I have this problem.

Such experiences of being discredited or ignored or devalued in any way, either intentionally or unintentionally, contributes to the isolation of the ill person and may affect the carer as well, as it did for Gary and his wife. There is always a possibility that the suffering extends to family members. As nurses and caring professionals we must not lose sight of this possibility.

The relationship between the ill person and their lay carer/s is likely to be altered because of the illness. It is not unusual that the ill person feels they are a burden on others:

> I was feeling really sort of down because I was thinking 'what a burden I am'. I sort of felt hopeless. That I wasn't doing enough.

These feelings often feed the suffering of that person, as their loss of independence may be accompanied by a sense of guilt and shame, and may even lead to a sense of reduced self-worth. It requires that those in caring roles have realistic expectations of the person with the illness, to ensure that they do not become impatient and hence further diminish the sufferer's self-worth, and disrupt their relationship with the sufferer (Charmaz 1983). Expectations range from being involved in household chores, social activities, intimate relationships and other responsibilities.

Whilst waiting for an appointment with Gary on one occasion, his wife took the opportunity to talk to the nurse. She felt, as a spouse, unsupported by health care professionals yet, as she pointed out, it was she who 'carries' Gary, as well as picking up a large share of his normal work. She felt devalued, unacknowledged and unappreciated for the substantially increased responsibilities brought to bear by Gary's dialysis dependency. She contrasted Gary's jovial behaviour and 'being the life of the party' whenever in the renal unit, to his 'grumpy' nature when at home. She indicated that she resented working the majority of the twelve hours, Monday to Friday, in their small business, as well as time over the weekends, as well as maintaining their home and caring for their children, whilst Gary 'would come and go as he pleased'.

While families are caught up in the suffering of a loved one, moving through the suffering is in many ways an individual experience. To resolve suffering, individuals work towards making sense of the experience, drawing meaning from it. Reality seeps in and over time the person becomes more focused, moving from the event (past), through the emotions (present) towards a future. Ill individuals attempt to maintain their self-worth and value in order to preserve themselves. Some sufferers may return to uncertainty if a goal is identified with no means to achieve it. Suffering however has the potential to transform through the opportunities of growth and discovery—by self-transcendence, getting outside the self or rising above the self, or setting a goal and accomplishing it, beyond the expectation of self and/or others, or by experiencing the good and beautiful in one's life, which is considered precious or by the attitude one takes to find some meaning in the illness.

Gary identified how some of the others in the renal unit got through their suffering. He noted that some people saw how they could help others in the same position by talking to them; one person saw dialysis as her 'job' three times a week; a few believed in God and that belief got them through; another decided she didn't want to be a complainer so made a decision to get on with her life; another decided that he was not going to let dialysis beat him and he continued his work and even got a promotion. For Gary, a desire to help others was important:

> If you can help one person down the road, like someone has helped me. If you can repay it with just one person you know, you have done something. It makes it better somehow.

At this juncture in the chapter, it would be clear to you that the emotional and physical suffering associated with illness can be profound, and those living with illness, chronic or acute, may experience significant challenges. Sometimes these challenges are so daunting that a person's quality of life is radically affected, and life may not seem worth living.

Yet you may know people who, despite these difficulties and illnesses, manage well and seem to enjoy life. Despite the obvious negative consequences of illness, there may, over time, be positive outcomes for some. These outcomes include personal growth, strength, increased spiritual convictions, altered values and visions and a recognition of being nurtured by others through this time. For some, then, 'suffering is a process of repair' (Morse & Penrod 1999, p 148).

Gary had this to say about getting on with life:

> I am not even busting my guts to get a kidney transplant because I know that it is going to take time. If it turns up tomorrow you are laughing, but if it doesn't you just have to wait. It is something to look forward to. I still think 'why me?', but not to the same anguish as in the past. I accept that it is me and compared to a lot of other people, I'm pretty well. It could have got a lot worse and I'm better off than many.

Gary's words suggest that he has managed to find an emotional pathway through his suffering. He acknowledges that he still suffers, but says this is not as intense as it used to be.

How do people survive emotionally through this kind of suffering? What is it that helps them to deal with pain, fatigue, changes to body image, uncertainty and so on? This second half of the chapter will help you to answer that question.

# Resilience

Resilience is a term used to describe the capacity to move through and beyond adversity. That some individuals who have experienced adversity actually do well despite their experiences suggests that there are no simple cause and effect relationships between negative experiences and levels of emotional distress. Instead, there are factors that assist the individual to survive and successfully resolve difficult life experiences.

There has been a growing focus on studying resilience over the past twenty-five years, and on related concepts such as invulnerability, growth, protective factors, stress-resistance, competence, meaning-making, coping and social support. This is illustrative of a move from a deficit-vulnerability model to a strengths perspective that explains why many people are able to deal with adversity (Lam & Grossman 1997). Studying resilience is popular because it allows those working in health-related disciplines 'to inject some hope and optimism into the dispiriting story of stress and adversity' (Rutter 1987, p 316). A problem-based perspective offers little insight into the nature of successful living, and does not explain how some individuals are able to withstand pressures that so profoundly affect the emotional and physical health of others.

Rutter (1987) suggested that resilience could be thought of as the opposite of vulnerability, with a continuum between the two. The degree to which an individual is resilient is likely to vary across a lifetime, often in relation to changing environmental circumstances. Whereas individuals may respond well to a particular stressor, they may succumb to another.

Resilience suggests a complex personal strength in the face of adversity (Lam & Grossman 1997). Does this mean that a resilient person meets all stressors with equanimity and personal equilibrium, as well as courage? What about a person who succumbs to grief, anger and/or depression in response to a trauma, such as being diagnosed with a life-threatening illness, or living with chronic pain?

In reality, resilience is not an 'all or nothing quality'. Developing resilience may be a process that takes many years of personal work. Gary's story provides us with evidence of this: he describes very eloquently just how much he suffered, yet he also describes getting through that suffering to a point where he says:

> It could have got a lot worse and I'm better off than many.

Being resilient may mean acknowledging personal difficulties and working to overcome them, rather than having no difficulties at all. It is highly likely, then, that a resilient person may not always be strong in the face of adversity, but may struggle over time to develop the resources to move beyond their particular trauma.

Focusing on resilience offers nurses and other caring professionals the opportunity to move beyond the illness model and focus on wellness (Polk 1997, Wagnild & Young 1990). Focusing on how people overcome health-related difficulties helps us to identify strategies for coping, which we can then share with those patients and their families who are in the early stages of their illness journey.

For example, nursing researchers in one qualitative study about resilience as people age (Wagnild & Young 1990) asked older women how they 'got through' difficult times. The major themes describing these women's responses to adversity were equanimity, perseverance, self-reliance, meaningfulness and existential aloneness. In other words, the women felt that accepting both the joys and sorrows of living, persisting even when facing adversity or being discouraged, having faith in oneself, having a purpose in life, and realising that life's journey is inevitably a solitary path helped them to journey through the more difficult times.

This notion was supported by another study about resilience in widowed women and men. McCrae & Costa (1988) found that, over time, recovery from bereavement meant that most of their participants did not live with any long-term psychosocial difficulties related to their loss. In other words, they had learnt to live with their loss and moved on with their lives. This was true in relation to self-related health, activities of daily living, size of their social network, communicating with others, psychological wellbeing, and their openness to new experiences. In each of the studies reviewed above, there was a recognition that learning had occurred as a consequence of the trauma. In other words, resilience was enhanced in the face of the adversity.

Using a different approach, Klohnen, Vandewater & Young (1996) argued that resiliency as a personal quality developed over time is a powerful resource that allows individuals to meet life challenges. In their study, women who were more resilient as they entered their middle years (assessed by observer ratings and self-report) reported greater levels of life satisfaction, better marital quality, more work satisfaction and better health throughout their middle years than those who were assessed as having lower resilience. This suggests that older people, with a variety of life experiences, may have learnt to deal with life's difficulties, and this then helps them face challenges more successfully.

## Resilience through illness

As we have argued, moving through illness can often bring about experiences that actually enhance quality of life over time, as well as a recognition of the positives from which the person with illness can draw strength and wisdom. For example, one recent Australian study detailing the experiences of long-term breast cancer survivors found that being diagnosed with, and treated for, breast cancer was a massive assault on both body and mind (Rogers-Clark 2002). Although the participants in this study described deep physical and emotional suffering, which for a number left deep and life-long scars, they also described a sense of renewed wonder about life, and a deeper appreciation for it.

How did they get to this point? Participants were asked this question, and responded by describing a number of personal responses which helped them to get through, which Rogers-Clark (2002) summarised under the following headings: 'doing', 'being determined', 'drawing strength from others', 'faith', 'being positive', and 'being inventive'.

The strategies that Gary used to move through his illness experiences bear many similarities to those found in the 2002 Rogers-Clark study, and are discussed below.

### Doing

Those living with illness have said that being active in the face their illness is a resilient response that has helped them to deal emotionally with their health crisis (Rogers-Clark 2002). For some, 'doing' involves being proactive with treatment, which helps them to feel more in control of their health. For others, 'doing' involves focusing on their caring role, such as looking after children or elderly partners or relatives, or returning to work, at least in some capacity. For others 'doing' involves focusing on activities such as gardening and craft, which are a welcome diversion from the difficulty of their situation:

> For a while I did nothing. I let my wife take over the business. But after a while that didn't work. She got too tired, for one thing. So I decided to get involved again. The dialysis unit said I could go on afternoon dialysis, so my mornings were free, which is the busiest time in the shop. That made a big difference. I didn't have so much time to sit around and mope.

### Being determined

Being determined is another aspect of resilience, and was described as being important by long-term cancer survivors (Rogers-Clark 2002). It means staying focused on survival, and not entertaining the thought of an early death. Being determined also means simply keeping going:

> I'm pretty bloody-minded, you know. I wasn't gonna let this get the better of me. I'm determined to survive . . . I'm not ready to curl my toes up just yet.

### Drawing strength from others

Drawing strength from others can also be of real help in the journey through illness. Valuing close relationships as well as broader social networks is the essence of the relational pattern of resilience identified by Polk (1997). This includes being able to confide in another, derive comfort from another, associate with positive role models and seek out confidantes. Social support helps to reduce the incidence of anxiety and depression following diagnosis, and assists the survivor to bear the physical and emotional pain because she or he does not feel alone, but instead feels loved (Breaden 1998, Carter 1996, Roux 1993):

> I can talk all I like about me being a tough person, and that's why I've coped with this thing, but honestly that's not it. I couldn't cope with any of this without my wife, and the nurses and others in the dialysis unit. They get me through. They cheer me up when I'm down, they listen to me, and they put up with me. What more could you want?

### Faith

Faith is often seen as a core component in religion, but can also be related to believing in medicine and nursing, believing in self and believing in the healing properties of the environment. Faith in medicine is often particularly important, since medical treatment is seen as the major 'line of defence' against illness. LaTour (1996) described this as 'doctor bonding', in which there is hope that medical intervention will treat, and even cure, cancer and other serious illnesses. Faith in self refers to a feeling of self-confidence about one's capacity to get through difficulties, whilst faith in one's environment relates to being in the healing properties of places which promote a sense of peace and healing, such as being at home or being out in nature:

> You've just got to have faith. You've got to have faith in yourself, and you've got to have faith in the doctors and nurses. They know what they're doing and I think they're great people. I feel really confident with them.

Faith also relates to spiritual beliefs. Spirituality is concerned with 'consciousness, especially the experience of a larger, more expansive consciousness than our normal experience' (Winter 1996, p 293). Spirituality can provide connection with a domain somehow greater than the personal life, with which people are able to connect and be sustained through difficult times. For some, spirituality is explored and expressed through a spiritual tradition, such as Buddhism, Taoism, Christianity, Islam (Winter 1996). For others, their spirituality will be expressed through spiritually based practices such as yoga, or through personal contemplation and life choices. For those who are ill, spirituality can provide comfort, meaning and direction:

> I never was much of a one for religion. Sometimes the hospital chaplain comes and talks to me when I'm on the machines, and I feel better about things after those chats. He reckons having faith in something has got to be better than believing in nothing, and I'm starting to think he's right . . . not that I'd tell him that!

### Being positive

Being positive refers to a personal attitude of looking for the positives in every experience, even those that appear to be overwhelmingly negative. Personal beliefs such as valuing self-knowledge and reflection, having a positive view of the future, and finding positive meaning in experiences are examples of this resilient response (Polk 1997). A sense that life has a purpose, is worthwhile and meaningful, and that one's own life can make a valuable contribution, is also evidence of this pattern:

> If you can help one person down the road, like someone has helped me. If you can repay it with just one person you know, you have done something. It makes it better somehow.

Rogers-Clark (2002) identified three ways in which the participants in her study demonstrated a positive approach to their illness. These included believing that they would have a good outcome in terms of their illness; focusing on their 'luck' in staying alive when others around them with similar illnesses had died; and using humour as a way of dealing with difficult aspects of the illness experience. The women saw themselves as lucky (because they had survived whilst others had not), and it was this interpretation which appeared to support them through their emotional as well as physical recovery. It helped them to focus on the good things that had come out of their illness, like a renewed appreciation for life, and a realisation of what was important to them, and what was not:

> I'm different now. I used to worry about little things, but now I don't. I've looked death in the face and, believe me, life is a pretty good alternative. Each morning I read the obituary notices in the paper, and it's great seeing that I'm not listed! Every day is a good day because I'm here.

### Inventiveness

Inventiveness was the final aspect of resilience mentioned by the participants in the Rogers-Clark study (2002). This involved finding innovative ways around the practical problems associated with illness. It is often these problems that can be most challenging, and are likely to involve dealing with physical health issues. For example, changes in body shape, such as the loss of a breast following mastectomy, or a swollen abdomen from dialysis fluid, need to be accommodated, and perhaps hidden. People may choose to wear, for example, loose clothing to hide such changes. These strategies are often developed over time, and with experience. Listening to others with similar problems is good, because these strategies can be shared:

> I've always liked a beer with me mates. But I can't drink too much fluid because being on dialysis means I'm on fluid restrictions. So now I drink Scotch! It's got a good kick, too!

# Survivorship

There is a strong connection between resilience and survivorship. Survivorship is about living with adversity, and this is made possible by the use of resilient responses to deal with that adversity. These resilient responses are individualised, and are drawn from and enabled within the context of a person's life.

Lifton (1967) defined a survivor as 'one who comes into contact with death in some bodily or psychic fashion and has himself *(sic)* remained alive' (p 479). The term 'survivor' is also commonly used to describe those who have lived through life traumas such as being in a concentration camp, experiencing domestic violence, sexual abuse, and living with cancer. The survivor may have no other choices available than to try to survive but can never be sure of this outcome.

An important distinction to be made when considering those who must face terrible life ordeals is between victims and survivors. A victim is powerless, whereas a survivor is someone who will take some control, regardless of how tenuous that may be (Merritt-Gray & Wuest 1995). Des Pres (1976) argued that survivors have a faith in themselves that allows them to find and use whatever small shred of power is available to them, no matter how despairing their situation might be. For example, Gary spoke about his friend Mary, who had advanced breast cancer but elected not to have chemotherapy because she wanted whatever time she had left to be quality time. She spoke of having a full life, filled with children and grandchildren, and she said she had reached a point where she was satisfied with her life. She was aware of the consequences of her choice, but felt she was choosing life and death on her own terms, and with the loving support of her husband. She had no control over the inevitability of her impending death, but she was able to make choices about how she wished to respond to it.

# Supporting people through suffering and developing resilience: Role of nurses

Whatever meaning is drawn by individuals about suffering, it exists and sufferers deserve relief and support. The first requirement is that suffering needs to be recognised. Although this sounds obvious, an evaluative process is required by nurses. Most often we assume suffering in another because we would suffer in the same circumstances. This may be a false compassion (Cassell 1991, p 31):

> It is sadly true that people are often insensitive to the suffering of others and when they do assign it a category it is frequently incorrect and self-serving.

Thus, a more systematic approach is warranted to ensure that nurses are open and sensitive to whether a patient is suffering. To really listen is one of the most helpful things a nurse can do. Good listeners listen with their heart as well as their ears. They are able to read between the lines and interpret unspoken non-verbal communications. To be a good listener, it is important to be focused completely on the other person, listen to *how* they are saying it as well as *what* they are saying. Nurses should be aware that people suffering may be afraid to say how they are feeling for fear that they will be thought of negatively. It is important to mobilise the sufferer's inner resources by using constructive, carefully chosen words, in the context of a caring relationship. Compassion can be a powerful activator of healing resources, but only if it is genuine. Most importantly, nurses must not lose sight of the fact that each person will experience illness and suffering in their own way for, without such recognition, sufferers may feel as if they are thought of as a body with a disease rather than a unique human being.

As nurses we need to ensure that we do not deflect the focus of attending to a person's suffering by focusing on what they are 'suffering from'. The latter moves the focus to a pathological emphasis, one where we can observe and measure. Instead we need to ensure that suffering is not relegated to the 'too hard' basket that inevitably compounds the experience of suffering. Instead, nurses need to focus on the whole person and what gives them a sense of completeness, identity and purpose.

When the sufferer reaches out for help and support, the provision of hope can be a lifeline. Hope can be provided by sharing stories of other survivors who have met and responded positively to the challenges now confronting the sufferer. This might be in the context of a support group, or via membership of an online discussion group.

The journey through suffering is rarely linear. Nurses should avoid expectations of a 'normal' timeframe and process of emotional or physical healing. This point is highlighted in Chapter 10, Living with Loss and Grief, but is worth noting again here. Those who continue to suffer, and appear not to be developing resilience, are most in need of our empathy and support. Accepting that a person may find the hurdles of their chronic illness insurmountable is the first step in helping that person, since it is impossible to be empathic when there is a belief that the person who is suffering should be 'getting over it'.

In the short term, medications to treat anxiety and depression may provide some welcome relief for the sufferer, and hence their use may be warranted. However, the danger with the use of such medications is that they may be used without resort to other healing modalities, such as counselling and ongoing support. Used in such ways, they serve only as a 'prop' to the person who is suffering, and are unlikely to provide any long-term solutions to their distress.

For those whose suffering is overwhelming, the assistance of a specialist nurse counsellor, psychologist or social worker may indeed be most helpful in assisting them to work through their feelings, and consider new strategies for responding to these. However, this approach will fail if those who continue to suffer deeply gain the impression that nurses and other health professionals have 'given up' on them.

## Conclusion

Confronting illness is perhaps one of the most significant life challenges a person is likely to confront. As with every other new situation, it is common for those newly diagnosed to feel overwhelmed and out of control. Normal life patterns may be changed irrevocably, and there may be a sense of overwhelming loss that elements of the individual's previous life are forever gone. The ensuing emotional suffering may overshadow any physical pain associated with the illness.

Fortunately, humans are adaptable beings. In the face of adversity, resilience begins. Perhaps it is slow at first, but for many who face chronic illness, eventually that illness is incorporated and managed within their daily lives. Life as they knew it may have changed, but that change is accommodated and the positive things in their new life are identified and cherished. At times, there is likely to be a return to suffering, where hope is lost, but here again resilience is likely to help the individual move through that particular chasm.

Nurses have much to learn from those who live with illness, and those who are wise will listen carefully. People who have learnt to live with a chronic illness can be excellent role models for those newly commenced on their illness journeys, and have much to offer those of us who would wish to care for them.

## Tutorial questions

1. Imagine you were diagnosed with end-stage renal disease and that you needed to have dialysis three times a week at the local hospital. Consider, and write down, the likely impact of this disease, and its treatment, on your current life.

   a) How do you think you would cope?

   b) How would you want to be treated by nurses?

2. This chapter focuses heavily on people who learn to accommodate their illness in their lives. What about people who seem to be overwhelmed and unable to move forward. How could you help in this situation?

## References

Breaden K 1998 Cancer and beyond: the question of survivorship. *Journal of Advanced Nursing* 26(5):978–984

Cassell E 1991 *Recognizing Suffering*. Hastings Center Report, May–June, pp 24–31

Carter BJ 1996 Understanding the experiences of long-term survivors of breast cancer: Story as a way of knowing. In: KH Dow (ed), *Contemporary Issues in Breast Cancer*. Jones and Bartlett, Boston

Charmaz K 1983 Loss of self: a fundamental form of suffering in the chronically ill. *Sociology* 5(2):168–195

Dewar A, Morse J 1995 Unbearable incidents: failure to endure the experience of illness. *Journal of Advanced Nursing* 22:957–964

Des Pres T 1976 *The Survivor: An Anatomy of Life in the Death Camps*. Oxford University Press, New York

Kleinman A 1991 Pain and resistance: the delegitimation and relegitimation of local worlds. In: M Good, P Brodwin, B Good, A Kleinman (eds) *Pain as human experience: an anthropological perspective*. University of California Press, Berkeley, pp 1–28

Klohnen EC, Vandewater EA Young A 1996 Negotiating the middle years: ego-resiliency and successful midlife adjustment in women. *Psychology and Ageing* 11(3):431–442

Lam JN, Grossman FK 1997 Resiliency and adult adaptation in women with and without self-reported histories of childhood sexual abuse. *Journal of Traumatic Stress* 10(2):175–196

LaTour K 1996 The breast cancer journey and emotional resolution: a perspective from those who have been there. In: KH Dow (ed), *Contemporary Issues in Breast Cancer*. Jones and Bartlett, Boston, pp 131–150

Lifton RJ 1967 *Death In Life: The Survivors of Hiroshima*. Weidenfeld and Nicholson, London

McCrae RR, Costa PT 1988 Psychological resilience among widowed men and women: a 10 year follow up of a national sample. *Journal of Social Issues* 44(3):129–142

Merritt-Gray M, Wuest J 1995 Counteracting abuse and breaking free: the process of leaving revealed through women's voices. *Health Care for Women International* 16:399–412

Morse J 1997 Responding to threats to integrity of self. *Advances in Nursing Science* 19(4):21–25

Morse J, Penrod J 1999 Linking concepts of enduring, uncertainty, suffering and hope. Image: *Journal of Nursing Scholarship* 31(2):145–150

Polk LV 1997 Toward a middle-range theory of resilience. *Advances in Nursing Science* 19(3):1–13

Rogers-Clark C 2002 *Resilient Survivors: Rural Women Who Have Lived Through Breast Cancer.* Doctoral Dissertation, University of Southern Queensland, Australia

Roux GM 1993 *Phenomenologic Study: Inner Strength in Women with Breast Cancer.* Doctoral dissertation, Texas Woman's University

Rutter M 1987 Psychosocial resilience and protective mechanisms. *American Journal of Orthopsychiatry* 57(3):316–331

Wagnild G, Young HM 1990 Resilience among older women. *Image: Journal of Nursing Scholarship* 22(4):252–255

Winter D 1996 *Ecological Psychology: Healing the Split between Planet and Self.* Harper Collins, New York

# Chapter 12

## The Spiritual Dimension in Nursing Care

*Noel Schultz*

**This chapter:**

- describes what is meant by spirituality and spiritual wellbeing;
- illustrates how matters of the spirit and spiritual wellbeing have been presented in nursing literature;
- highlights the spiritual needs of persons with dementia and the contribution that nursing care can make to their spiritual wellbeing; and
- draws attention to the importance of preparation for effective involvement in the spiritual dimension of nursing care.

Within nursing, there is a growing interest in the role of the spiritual dimension as an important component of healing. The spiritual, together with the physical, the emotional, the social, and the psychological are integral to being human. Matters of the spirit are often of major importance when illness and other undesirable life transitions occur. At such times, added importance surrounds questions concerning one's identity, the meaning of life, one's relatedness to others, and the purposes suffering can serve. The search for peace of mind and the importance of hope (which are part of the human experience throughout life) now have added relevance.

This chapter provides an introduction to spirituality, especially as it relates to people who are ill, from a nursing perspective. The importance of seeking to define the meanings given to spirituality and the distinction that needs to be made between spirituality and religiosity preface a brief exploration of the spiritual dimension for persons with dementia. The extent to which nurses have a shared responsibility in addressing the spiritual concerns of dementia patients and how this might be approached are also considered. Using the example of dementia is relevant given the large numbers of Australians living with the illness, or caring for someone who does.

In nursing practice, interest in the spiritual continues to grow. The hospice movement has been a major contributor to this development (Barnum 1996, Chandler 1999), as has been a deepening commitment to holistic nursing. Both these influences have encouraged an exploration of the spiritual dimension as it relates to those who are ill and/or dying, and those who love them. Two other major contributors to the growing interest in the spiritual domain have been the New Age movement, with its links to Eastern spiritualities (Confoy 2002, Heelas 1996, Tacey 1997), and those areas of alternative medicines that include meditation and prayer (Brown-Saltzman 1997, Dossey 1993). All these contributors have led to an increased recognition amongst nurses of the importance of spiritual care as an important component of person-centred care (Carson 1989, Hutchison 1997, Sims 1987).

The current emphasis on the spiritual is not a religion-inspired phenomenon. In reality, the widespread acknowledgment that the spiritual is an area of life that has needs and potentials for health and wellbeing has come at a time when the Christian religion is in numerical decline in much of the Western world and its influence on the thought patterns of our day is greatly diminished. Confoy (2002) argued that there is widespread dissatisfaction with organised religions in answering spiritual concerns in today's world. Clearly, then, we need to look beyond today's religious institutions to understand the growing interest in the spiritual as an integral part of person-centred nursing care. Perhaps the scientific approach to health, life, death and what lies beyond, which has long maintained dominance in health care, is now becoming more open to the possibility that the spiritual may offer a supplementary contributor to human wellbeing.

# The person and spiritual wellbeing

Human beings, who are body–mind–spirit entities, have five dimensions with needs specific to each dimension:

1. the physical—with needs, for example, for food and fluids;
2. the social—with needs, for example, to relate, to love and be loved, to experience mutuality and friendship;
3. the emotional—with needs, for example, to experience and express feelings;
4. the psychological—with needs, for example, of security, comfort, safety; and
5. the spiritual—with needs to find a sense of purpose and meaning, hope, and peace of mind.

Spirit can be viewed as the central core of a person's being. When the spirit is healthy and whole, the flow of energy, or spiritual wellbeing, is integrated into the whole person so that the other dimensions of the person, the physical, social, emotional and psychological, are all enriched. Shamy (1997) claimed that the spiritual embraces the essence of what it means to be human, integrating and holding together the physical, psychological and social dimensions of life. Emotions, too, are profoundly influenced by the condition of a person's spirit. Anecdotal evidence has highlighted that it is not uncommon for those who have achieved inner peace and hope in a relationship of trust with others, to have an awareness of wholeness and healing even when there is no cure for physical aliments or when serious disabilities cause ongoing major difficulties to their lives.

Spiritual wellbeing, then, can be an integrating power for the person who is aware of his/her individual identity, not in isolation from but in relationship with others. This person is able to affirm life in its fullness within him/herself, in relationships with others, and in harmony with the environment and whoever or whatever is that person's highest good.

# What is meant by spirituality?

The spiritual is an integral part of being a person. In its broadest sense, spirituality is the manifestation of the human spirit, just as physiology is one manifestation of the body (Laukhuf & Werner 1998). The inner spirit of a person has needs, just as the person's body and mind does. There are diseases of the spirit, just as there are of the body. The spiritual is that dimension of a person that prompts questions like these:

- Does my life have meaning?
- Is there some power or being beyond what I can see?
- What are the perceptions that I have about life that influence my values?

From a nursing perspective, it is also important to consider why peace of mind, hope, and a sense of belonging appear to be important to human wellbeing and how these states of being can be obtained and retained. In my practice, I have noted that when a person feels 'together' and at peace within, then major transitions and undesirable experiences are not only survived, but can even become growth experiences. In a slightly different vein, it is interesting to consider what it is about some people that cause others in their presence to experience remarkable tranquility and a rekindling of hope.

Reed (1992) described spirituality as a person's capacity for self-transcendence, which allows that person to experience connectedness inter-personally, intra-personally, and trans-personally. It is also a personal, individual value system about the way people approach and view their life, in relationship with others and in the face of life's upheavals, changes, setbacks and opportunities. It is constantly evolving, developing, and perhaps contracting. At different stages in life, the focus may shift from one area of the spiritual domain to another. Thus, in the early years of life, the focus may tend to be on the search to establish one's own identity; in later years, more attention may be directed to such questions as 'Have I achieved my life goals? What are my hopes for the years that remain?'

While some writers are hesitant about attempting a definition of the spiritual, since it is an individual matter and has a mystical element to it, there have been numerous attempts at seeking to define the meaning of spirituality especially as it relates to nursing and other health care workers. Definitions of spirituality include the following: seeks meaning (May 1982); connectedness to self, others and a higher being (Burkhardt & Nagai-Jacobson 2002); focus to our living and loving (Confoy 2002); and is present in all individuals as a relationship with a transcendent God or supreme reality and is manifested as inner peace and strength (Narayanasamy 1999).

# Human spirituality and wellbeing

Who one is, one's 'self', refers to our perceptions of who we are, which we are able to assess through relationships with others, the environment, and with 'the other' (however understood). In relationships, for example, we are often confronted with the best and worst in ourselves, sometimes in the form of direct feedback from those we relate to. Growing out of this process is the formation and shaping of a personal sense of identity. Being sure of one's identity is of particular importance at various stages in life's journey; for example, when separating from parents, when engaging in deep reciprocal relationships, when facing major transitions, when experiencing dramatic losses or when confronted by life-threatening illnesses.

For each individual there is a need to have some purpose to live in order to perceive a satisfying and fulfilling life. The acquired meanings and purpose that we give to our lives may be challenged when we encounter tragedy, losses and changes beyond our control in our lives. It is during these times that we may examine what is beyond the self, others and the environment, beyond all that we have known and seek some higher power to be able to vision its meaning in a new light. We may well seek to understand the nature of this other, this power, force, mind, spirit, or god and how to transcend our worldly reality.

The spirit seeks to integrate values and to espouse special qualities. It is aware of the importance to the self of hope and of being at peace within one's self and with others. It recognises a responsibility of care for the environment and the importance of helping others to experience justice, and the opportunity to experience holistic wellbeing. The spirit also seeks to nurture and sustain both self and others by engaging fully in life, through creative activities, and through the embracing of beauty, truth, and the majesty of the universe. The spirit treasures moments of transcendence and mystery.

# Religion and spirituality

As noted earlier in this chapter, spirituality is not synonymous with religion or belief in a god, but is something much broader. Laukhuf & Werner (1998, p 61) explain this distinction:

> Religion is the service and adoration of God or a god expressed in forms of worship. Religion refers to the external formalised system of beliefs whereas spirituality is concerned with a personal interpretation of life and the inner resource of people.

Spirituality is a dimension of and has importance in the lives of persons of all cultures, of all faiths, and of no faiths. Religion as distinct from spirituality is more about systems of practice and beliefs, rituals and community engagement. Religion can provide a platform for the expression of one's spirituality, but religious beliefs and practices can also discourage a development of the spiritual dimension (Dyson, Cobb & Forman 1997). This can occur when religious beliefs become blinding dogma, and rituals are blindly followed without a continuing focus on the key spiritual messages underpinning such beliefs and practices.

In formal religious practices, such as prayer, meditation, worship, compassionate and charitable behaviours, many do, however, discover that these expressions of their religiosity are vital ways for the ongoing development of their spirit life. Likewise, it is through religious beliefs about a god and the person's relationship to this 'other' and to the special persons in their world that many religious practitioners discover wholeness, health, and a rich life.

Many influences are at work in shaping a person's spirituality. The predominant religious culture surrounding a person—whether it is Christianity, Judaism, Buddhism, Islam, Shintoism, Hinduism, Confucianism or Taoism, in one or more of their various expressions—will be one contributing factor to the person's responses to spiritual considerations. There are many other influences on spirituality, including educational experiences, the stimulation provided by a variety of cultures, exposure to the arts, and attitude towards nature, to name a few. Consequently even for people engaged in a satisfying religious framework in which they express important aspects of their spirituality, such religiosity is not their only route to spiritual wellbeing. Persons from similar cultures and religious environments will frequently express their spirituality in different ways and find support for the spiritual dimension in their lives through different means, such as music, meditation, community service, corporate worship or gardening.

With this broad understanding of the spiritual dimension the next section of this chapter considers the spiritual needs and concerns of persons who are ill.

# Spiritual care and nursing practice

Laukhuf & Werner (1998, p 67) describe spiritual care as an integral part of good nursing practice:

> Spiritual care involves the caring practices we exhibit as nurses. It takes the guise of those practices we do daily that affect our patient's spirit in profound ways. Spiritual care is more than realizing a patient's spiritual beliefs and incorporating them into our interventions. Spiritual care is anything that touches the spirit of another. It can be shared laughter, tears, or remembering their birthday. It can be keeping vigil with that family when the patient dies. It can be soothing chronically-ill individuals as they struggle to define their worth and meaning in the face of illness and other demands, or it can be as simple as just sitting there . . . Spiritual care is not provided only for those who believe a certain way or who define God by a specific doctrine. Spiritual care is for everyone. People express their spirituality in unique ways. Everyone has a spiritual nature that can be touched through the ministrations of another.

In seeking to understand and address the spiritual needs and concerns of persons, the intention is to contribute to the healing of the patient, not necessarily the curing. As discussed in Chapter 2, persons can and do experience healing even when their physical illness continues. Thus, nursing care embraces spirituality when that care assists the patient to make sense of their situation, to find meaning or purpose in their day and in relationships, to reframe the past, to receive approval and acceptance and to know they are loved and can give love (Kirkland & McIlveen 1999, p 246).

Our case study considers the experiences of Mary, who has dementia. An individual who is cognitively impaired continues to be a person with needs in the physical, social, spiritual, psychological, and emotional dimensions of his/her personhood, even when the ability to express those needs clearly has diminished.

# Case study

Mary was diagnosed by her medical practitioner as suffering from dementia. She was 68 years of age, married to Jack who was seven years her senior, the mother of two sons, and the grandmother of five girls. An 18-year-old daughter had died following a car accident. Mary and her husband had lived most of their lives in a provincial city where Jack had been the owner/manager of a small business. Both had maintained a deeply spiritual outlook on life—they attended their church regularly, and were regarded as people of strong religious faith.

When Mary and Jack became aware that Mary's initial forgetfulness was developing to a stage where both were concerned, they shared their fears with one another and faced the possibility that it was the early stages of dementia. Mary was inclined not only to forget what day it was, how to use the washing machine and the names of her granddaughters, but also how to prepare a simple meal and how to dress herself. Mary and Jack had been planning a major round-the-world trip when Mary's illness forced a major rethink of their future plans.

Their attendance at religious observances became infrequent. Mary found much of it incomprehensible, and Jack wanted to protect his wife from any embarrassment. For five years after the illness was diagnosed, Mary was cared for at home by her devoted husband. For them dementia was a most undesirable but unavoidable invasion into their lives. They had informed themselves on the particular dementia and had made plans for the years ahead. They talked openly about the reality that Mary would never be healed, that her condition would inevitably deteriorate, but they helped each other to adapt to the reality. Mary had confidence that her husband would continue to support her and treat her with love and respect as a person of worth even when she no longer knew him or who she was. In her spirit she knew herself to be loved and at peace.

Towards the end of this period, Jack's health began to deteriorate. He was assisted by the weekly visit of a community nurse. Jack and Mary discovered with relief that the nurse quickly perceived that here was a couple who knew healing when no cure was possible. A long-time friend of Mary and Jack who was a volunteer pastoral care worker from their church, continued his regular visits, prayed with them and celebrated the Eucharist with them.

# Living with Illness

Dementia is a common illness. More than 162,000 Australians currently have dementia (Access Economics 2003). A collection of symptoms found in many dementia patients include impairment of memory, inability to learn new information, or to retain past personal information, or facts of common knowledge. Impairment of two or more brain functions, including memory, language, cognitive skills, emotional behavior, personality and visual–spatial perceptions suggest the presence of dementia (Boden 2000). There are no cures for dementia, but early and correct diagnosis and medication can help stabilise the condition.

With the onset of dementia, the patient comes face to face with questions that are at the heart of spirituality. A profound sense of what has already been lost and the enormity of what will inevitably and progressively be lost—never to be reclaimed—is the grim reality that confronts the dementia patient. As dementia progresses, patients will lose a sense of their own identity, and the people who were previously central to life will become strangers to them. With loss of memory it will become increasingly difficult to frame their present in the context of past years. With progressive damage to the brain, the person is unable to meet their own needs because their cognitive capacity progressively deteriorates. The fact that the former integration of body, mind, and spirit is being progressively destroyed strikes at the very core of a person's being.

In seeking to provide care to a person with dementia, it is quickly apparent what the patient has lost. It is an understandable response to focus on these losses, yet it is much more productive to become aware of and to use what has not been lost to the person than to deplore the deficits (Schultz 2004, Shamy 1997).

## Case study ... *continued*

Following Jack's death, Mary was quickly admitted to a nursing home in her city. She grieved deeply for the husband she had loved from early adulthood. For six months she was totally confused in her unfamiliar environment. Male doctors were often greeted as though they were her husband. Female nurses were seen by Mary as her 18-year-old daughter who had died in an accident 50 years previously. The gentle Mary of earlier years was now at times abusive and aggressive. Profound sadness, totally unrelated to what was happening around her, characterised much of her behaviour.

There were other times, however, when there was obvious calm and peace within her spirit. At the weekly chapel service she shared in the prayers and hymns and even volunteered to play her favorite song. Though she was often not sure what her name was, she was able to say verses from the Psalms without prompting.

Mary and her husband had made some preparation for the time when aged care home accommodation would be needed. Knowing that his ill health was likely to lead to his death before Mary's, Jack had written *Mary's Story* in which he described in considerable detail her origins, her childhood, the experiences that brought special joy or sorrow, the flowers she loved, the perfume she used, the songs she enjoyed singing, the bible verses she treasured, the stories about her children and her friends that she was always ready to retell, the poems she learned by heart, the groups she belonged to and the part she played in her church and community. Photographs of Mary at important events throughout her life, with appropriate captions, featured prominently. This information enabled Mary's nurses to access Mary's world, and helped them and her family to remind her of who she was and all she had experienced in her life. Mary's story also often provided cues for Mary to express emotions. On increasingly rare occasions Mary surprised and delighted nurses when she talked briefly with lucidity of experiences from the past as well making comments about the here and now of her aged care environment.

# Challenges in caring for the spiritual needs of the patients

There are many challenges for a nurse endeavouring to incorporate care of a spiritual kind into the holistic care regime. For a start, there is the nurse's uncertainty about the spiritual area of his/her own life. This may arise out of confusion of spirituality with religiosity, or the equally mistaken notion that to be responsive to the spiritual needs and concerns of a patient a nurse has to use 'God-talk' and religious jargon, or to seek to direct the patient to representatives of a particular religious perspective or theology.

To provide nursing care that includes the spiritual, nurses are unable to rely on a scientific approach. Instead nurses must rely largely on their own insights, humanity and empathy when considering the spiritual domain of those they care for. It is very difficult to give that which one does not have oneself, so it is important that nursing students clarify what brings meaning to their own lives as part of their preparation for practice.

There are significant barriers to providing spiritual care. Nurses may fear being perceived as incompetent or feel uneasy if they believe they are unable to meet particular spiritual requests of patients, such as prayer. If nurses have not reflected on their own spiritual beliefs and values, they may find it difficult to know how to respond to another's spiritual needs or concerns. Perhaps the major barrier is a perception that spiritual care is a specialised area which nurses are not qualified to respond to. If nurses incorrectly assume that spirituality is a specifically religious concept, they may shift the responsibility of this form of care to others, such as chaplains and religious agents, and take the position that the spirituality needs of their patients are not their concern.

Some nurses may avoid spiritual issues because they are worried about imposing their own views or intruding on their patients' privacy. Yet, there is usually not the same concern when nurses intrude in patients' intimate space by implementing strategies which socially would normally be labelled as 'private', such as assessing elimination patterns and sexual habits.

Spiritual care stands in sharp contrast to the emphasis on 'doing' that tends to guide a good deal of contemporary health care practice. In the current climate, which emphasises 'outputs' and cost effectiveness, it can be difficult to find time to consider and incorporate nursing responses to patient's spiritual needs. A further challenge is the reducing numbers of registered nurses in relation to the number of patients, creating an environment where care may be more orientated to physical care, because that is all that can be achieved given staffing constraints.

These challenges are real and can be difficult to overcome. Yet this chapter has clearly demonstrated that true holistic care must include a focus on the spiritual domain of patients. If spiritual distress is not accurately identified, there is the possibility that treatment will be inappropriately directed by a biomedical and/or psychological and/or cultural domain. At times, spiritual interventions such as helping a person consider spiritual matters can indeed take a lot of time. This, however, is not always the case. More often, spiritual care is exemplified by an approach to everyday nursing tasks which values the sacred spirit of each person. This approach may well be no more time-consuming than providing care that lacks this spiritual emphasis. Nellie and Ruth demonstrated this type of spiritual caring when looking after Mary.

---

## Case study . . . *continued*

*Mary's Story* enabled Nellie and Ruth, two of her regular long-time nurses, to gain an understanding of Mary's grief but also of her hope, as well as cues to her sense of contentment. Whenever attending to Mary's physical needs, they never failed to address her as 'Mary', identified themselves as 'Nellie' or 'Ruth'. They ensured that Mary's visitors from the church community were given unimpeded access to Mary, introduced to her each time they came, and a record kept of their visits so that Mary's family could be assured that she was not being neglected. On warm days, a brief stroll around Mary's favorite section of the garden was enjoyed by Mary and her attending nurse. At the end of their shift, it was their practice to touch Mary's hand or forehead and say goodbye, repeating who they were and who Mary was. As Mary's condition deteriorated further and she was confined to bed, they continued to talk to Mary with respect and kindness, and on rare quiet times would sit by her bedside for a few moments and gently hold her hand. Nellie and Ruth and Mary's sons shared their insights and their feelings during the months leading up to her death. Nellie and Ruth were especially invited to her funeral and spoke with sincerity of their privilege in caring for Mary in the last years of her life. They referred to occasions when they had left her bedside without the stresses that were troubling them on entering her room. Something of Mary's spirit, of calmness and of quiet hope, had been imparted to them through being in her presence. They were convinced that deep within the inner recesses of Mary's being were assurances and hopes that were impossible to express.

---

Mary's experiences show that whilst spiritual care may not physically heal, it provides a graceful form of care when given to a person whose purpose and meaning in life has been challenged by illness. The case study demonstrates that spiritual care is a broad phenomenon, involving a range of nursing actions which might appear at first glance to have little direct relationship to spirituality, yet which have in common a respect for, and valuing of, the spiritual essence of a person. Nellie and Ruth demonstrated through their actions a continuing respect for Mary as a unique and worth-while person, despite the cognitive impairment and ensuing behaviours associated with her dementia. They understood the centrality of religious faith in Mary's life, and so encouraged the visits of members of Mary's church community as well as responding to the needs of Mary's family to know she was being well cared for. In so doing, they demonstrated their commitment to holistic nursing care.

# Conclusion

This chapter has considered the centrality of the spirit in the experience of being human. The concept of spirituality has been defined, and the differences between religiosity and spirituality explored. The importance of spiritual wellbeing to all humans, but especially to those who confront health-related difficulties has been acknowledged. Through a consideration of the spiritual needs of Mary, a woman with dementia, and the responses to these needs by Mary's nurses, key aspects of spiritual nursing care have been highlighted. This chapter has acknowledged that there are challenges in providing spiritual nursing care, but notes that responding to a patient's spiritual needs involves a broad range of responses which may be no more burdensome than providing nursing interventions without a spiritual emphasis.

# Tutorial questions

1. What gives your life meaning and purpose? Relate that to your under-standing of your own spirituality.

2. Discuss the following challenges to providing spiritual care for patients and identify ways in which the challenges might successfully be met:

   a) a nurse's uncertainty about the spiritual area in his/her own life;

   b) a nurse's belief that spirituality of a patient is private;

   c) difficulty in identifying when a patient's needs are spiritual; and

   d) when a patient' spiritual beliefs are different to those held by the nurse.

# References

Access Economics 2003 *The Dementia Epidemic: Economic Impact and Positive Solutions for Australia*. Access Economics, Canberra

Barnum B 1996 *Spirituality in nursing: From traditional to New Age*. Springer, New York

Boden C 2000 Ask us—the people with dementia—what we want. In: Dementia Forum Conference Proceedings, 16–17 August 1999, Aged and Community Care Division Department of Health and Aged Care, Commonwealth of Australia, Canberra, pp 29–36

# Living with Illness

Brown-Saltzman K 1997 Replenishing the spirit by meditative prayer and guided imagery. *Seminars in Oncology Nursing* 13:255–259

Burkhardt M, Nagai-Jacobson 2002 *Spirituality: Living our Connectedness.* Delmar/Thomson Learning, Albany, New York

Carson VB 1989 *Spiritual dimensions in nursing practice.* Saunders, Philadelphia

Chandler E 1999 Spirituality. In: Corless I, Foster Z (eds) *The Hospice Heritage: Celebrating our Future.* Haworth Press, New York, pp 63–74

Confoy M. 2002 The contemporary search for meaning in suffering. In: Rumbold BD (ed) *Spirituality and Palliative Care.* Oxford University Press, Melbourne, pp 22–37

Dossey L 1993 *Healing words: The power of prayer and the practice of medicine.* Harper Collins, New York

Dyson J, Cobb M, Forman D 1997 The meaning of spirituality: A literature review. *Journal of Advanced Nursing* 26:1183–1188

Heelas P 1996 The new age movement. Blackwell, Oxford

Hutchison MM 1997 Healing the whole person: The spiritual dimension of holistic care. Christian Nursing Page, marghut@ibm.net

Kirkland K, McIlveen H 1999 Full circle: Spiritual therapy for people with dementia. *American Journal of Alzheimer's Disease* 14:245–247

Laukhuf G, Werner H 1998 Spirituality: The missing link. *Journal of Neuroscience Nursing* 30:60–67

May GG 1982 *Will and Spirit: A Contemplative Psychology.* Harper and Row, San Francisco

Narayanasamy A 1999 A review of spirituality as applied to nursing. *International Journal of Nursing Studies* 36:117–125

Reed PG 1992 An emerging paradigm for the investigation of spirituality in nursing. *Research in Nursing and Health* 15:349–357

Schultz N 2004 *Forgetting but not forgotten: Understanding, support and spiritual care for persons with dementia and those who care for them.* Openbook, Adelaide

Shamy E 1997 *More than body, brain, and breath: A guide to spiritual care of people with Alzheimer's disease and related dementia.* ColCom Press Orewa, NZ

Sims C 1987 Spiritual care as part of holistic nursing. *Imprint* 34:63–65

Tacey D 1997 *Australia—in search of a soul.* Eremos, Parramatta

# Chapter 13

## Empowering Partnerships: Nurses and Those They Care For

*Kristine Martin-McDonald*

---

**This chapter:**

- explores the traditional roles of nurses and those they care for;
- discusses the concepts of empowerment and partnerships as they apply to the provision of health care;
- examines the key concepts of a partnership model:
  - a) non-patronising empowerment;
  - b) collaborative decision making;
  - c) valuing diversity and individuality; and
  - d) mutually beneficial relationship; and
- identifies the threat to each characteristic of the partnership model.

In this, the final chapter of this text, we discuss how nurses can effectively form healing partnerships with those they care for. Once nurses are able to appreciate the broad range of issues surrounding the illness experience, they can then consider approaches to working in partnership with their patients, aimed at enhancing the health and wellbeing of these patients. This chapter briefly examines the traditional roles of nurses and patients, before considering the characteristics of an empowering relationship, built on partnership. This kind of relationship requires a commitment to the notion that people who are ill and in need of health care should be in charge of their own care, with nurses working with them rather than taking control. The specific elements of partnership models—non-patronising empowerment, collaborative decisions and mutually beneficial outcomes—are discussed as well as the threats to each of the elements being implemented. Throughout this chapter a case study is presented to highlight the main points raised.

The notion of the sick patient as helpless, passive and reliant on the advice of health care professionals has been extensively challenged. In its stead is an approach that acknowledges the need for active involvement of patients in their care as well as in the development, implementation and evaluation of health policies and systems. The recipients of health care are increasingly seen as consumers, a move which is accompanied by a greater focus on patient rights (Germov 1999). Individuals are encouraged to take greater responsibility for their health and wellbeing, and easier access to health information means that the recipients of health care are often very well informed about their illness. As a result there has been a significant move to ensure a collaborative effort is fostered between the key stakeholders in the provision of health care, namely users of health services and the health professionals caring for them.

## Evolution of caring for the unwell

The most common term for the people that health professionals care for is 'patient'. 'Patient' has its origin in the Latin terms *patiens* and *pati* which means 'to suffer', 'one who suffers'. It is also used to define 'one that is actuated upon or undergoes an action' and 'one who receives medical attention, care or treatment' (Oxford Dictionary 2003). Historically the term 'patient' was associated with the sick role that Parsons (1950) described as legitimising a person's temporary exemption from normal social responsibilities whilst ill. Four assumptions underpinned this sick role:

1. The patient is exempt from usual roles and responsibilities.

2. The patient is not responsible for his or her incapacity (illness).

3. The patient is willing to get better (desire to leave this state of temporary incapacity or social deviance).

4. The patient is obliged to seek expert help and to cooperate with treatment regimes.

This designated sick role description has been criticised (Nyatanga & Dann 2002, Watt 2000). In these times there is more of an acceptance of diversity, blurring of role boundaries and an acknowledgment that individuals are unique. Those who are cared for by nurses are well positioned to know, understand and decide what is best in their life situation. If this is the case, then it would seem appropriate that each person ought to have the freedom to choose their behavioural options rather than be expected to conform to prescribed sick role behaviour.

## Case study

Jim is an active and healthy 67-year-old man who has been struggling to cope for a couple of years since the death of his wife. He explains to his son (Peter) that he has lost his 'zest' for life since then, and really has trouble getting interested in anything.

J:   I just can't be bothered, you know. Everything seems like too much of an effort.

P:   Have you seen anyone about this Dad?

J:      No! I'm not going to get treated like some mad idiot.

P:      But Dad, perhaps you need some help in managing how you're feeling right now. This problem won't disappear. There are some great nurses at the Community Mental Health Clinic. I know someone who went there for help, and she said it was great. Her nurse really listened to her, and asked her how she wanted to manage the problem.

J:      You mean a nurse might be interested in my opinion? The nurses in my day just told you what to do!

P:      Things have changed a lot in the last twenty years Dad.

J:      Yeah all right. I guess I've got nothing to lose.

Even the term 'patient' has been challenged as being inappropriate language for health care uses. The label 'patient' allows a mindset that renders the health professional superior to and in control of their patients (Nyatanga & Dann 2002). It is this traditional positioning of nurses that, if adopted, gives them significant control over their patients. In Jim's case, his previous experience with nurses was that they were always in the dominant position, and liked to keep things that way. Within this traditional model of nurse and patient, there can be some unfortunate consequences for 'patients' who ask questions, challenge the authority of the professionals or seek some control over the decisions related to their care. They might find that they are labelled as difficult and could be alienated for such behaviour. Some of the characteristics of both the nurse and the patient in this traditional model are identified in Table 1.

**Table 1:** Traditional Model of Health Care

### TRADITIONAL MODEL OF HEALTH CARE

| NURSE | PATIENT |
| --- | --- |
| Powerful | Powerless |
| Expert | Lay person |
| Prescribed care | Passive recipient |
| Language authoritative | Language accepting, respectful |
| Authoritative knowledge, training, skills in health matters | Lacks knowledge, skill in health matters |
| Narrow focus on care of disease or illness | Focus on getting well |
| Emotionally distant | Emotions kept in check |

This imbalance of power is problematic in relationships between nurses and health care users, particularly in relation to those who are chronically ill. Unlike acute illness, chronic illness by its definition is long-lasting. Whilst there is a diagnosis and treatment regimes, the tolerance of being exempted from social responsibilities, such as those given to people with acute illnesses, is short-lived for those with chronic illnesses. Chronic illnesses are managed rather than cured, may deteriorate over time, are often accompanied by additional diagnoses of other chronic illnesses, are unpredictable and diverse in their presentation in each person (Watt 2000). The focus in chronic illness is on delaying the progress of the disease, minimising acute exacerbations associated with the illness and maintaining optimal functioning for the individual for as long as is possible. Thus people with chronic illnesses are required to be self-managing, self-monitoring and largely self-treating.

Often those with chronic illness feel 'invisible' in the social world, particularly if they manage their illnesses well. This invisibility fails to validate the intrusiveness of the illness in all aspects of their lives and their families, and the need for constant vigilance and adaptation to the deterioration in the health of the sufferer. The changing face of the chronic illnesses continually challenges their image of who they are and what their place in the world is. The sick role fails to capture the experience of those living with chronic illness and the roles of their nurses (Watt 2000, p 14):

> In chronic conditions, providers normally hold little in the way of unique expertise and no curative ability. Therefore clinical decision-making is focused on disease management and the patient is not only empowered, but also often required, to take an active and central role in this process

# Empowerment

Despite improved medical technologies and long-term survivorship of chronic illnesses, modern medicine is heavily critiqued as being all-knowing and all-powerful as well as for its high costs (Germov 1999). The traditional roles of both nurses and those they care for continue to exist in health care settings, and in this context nurses might, wittingly or unwittingly, adopt ways of relating to those in their care which are intimidating to them. The hierarchical structure of many health care institutions and disciplines, supported through the use of the sick role model, is perhaps the most significant obstacle to empowered partnerships. Nyatanga & Dann (2000, p 237) hold a strong view that:

> As long as service users are referred to as patients and are expected to comply with the sick role then empowerment will remain an ideal that will never be realized.

Empowerment has Latin root origin in the word power, *potere*, which means 'to be able'. Its prefix 'em' means 'cause to be or provide with' (Oxford Dictionary 2003). Empowerment is seen as beneficial to the health of a person because it involves enhancing a person's capacity to influence or control significant aspects of their lives. Helping someone to be more empowered is about helping that person to develop the personal resources necessary to manage their own situation, rather than doing everything for them.

Empowerment requires recognition that both nurses and those they care for have expertise, which may differ in content and context but which, when assimilated, can be complementary. This has the potential to bring about the best health outcomes. Thus, if empowerment is to occur, nurses need to move out of their frame of reference as the expert. This does not imply that their expertise is not required or is obsolete, but rather requires a partnership approach where both nurses and users of their services come together for the benefit of the user.

Empowerment of patients has been advocated by the World Health Organization since 1986 (Houston & Cowley 2002) yet it remains somewhat elusive in health care settings (Tanner 1998, Ryles 1999). It has been argued that 'the acknowledged chink between ideals of user empowerment and realities of everyday practice is in fact a yawning chasm' (Tanner 1998, p 447) and that the 'subservient and deferential culture' of nursing (Ryles 1999, p 602) has created an unwillingness or inability to embrace empowerment.

## Case study . . . *continued*

Jim made an appointment with a mental health nurse at the clinic. Following the visit Jim and Peter talk.

P:  So how was it?

J:  You know he was really nice. He listened to me, and then talked about some different ways that we could work on the problem together. I really liked that. He says he thinks I'm depressed. He didn't use any of that fancy medical language, so I understood everything. He didn't push me to do what he thought was best either.

P.  So what are you going to do?

J.  I'm going back next week. The nurse says I can't expect to get better quickly, and he reckons it might be good if I also saw the psychiatrist at the clinic, to see if medication would help. I'm not sure about that one though. I'll stick with the nurse for now. It feels better just talking about things with him.

P:  Sounds good Dad.

Strategies for developing empowering partnerships with those we care for will differ according to the particular needs of each person. In Chapter 6, Multicultural Issues in Health, we are reminded of the enormous cultural differences in the perception of health and illness, and how important it is to ask those we care for to tell us about their cultural practices and beliefs. This is an important first strategy in ensuring culturally safe care. Consider also those from low socioeconomic status (SES) groups. Chapter 3, Class, Poverty and Chronic Illness—Intersecting Links, identifies that a key fact relevant to the poor health of lower SES workers is that they experience little control in their lives. With such a background it may be that these people bring an expectation that they will have no choice or say in their health care. Establishing empowering partnerships between nurses and disadvantaged or vulnerable minority groups may take time, special consideration and sensitivity to issues relevant to such groups.

We need to move from the ideal to the reality of empowerment to establish the foundation of an empowering partnership. Jim found himself actively involved in receiving information about the different types of treatment options for his depression. Jim's nurse did not use his expertise to create a gap between them. Instead the nurse frankly shared the relevant information using a language and manner that was respectful of Jim's level of understanding about his illness and treatment options. By doing so, the nurse demonstrated that he respected Jim, and valued his role in the decision-making process. It is all too easy for health care professionals to maintain an elite position by using medical jargon, a language that is foreign to most health care users. Empowerment means creating genuine opportunities, provision of encouragement and support, comprehensive information and presentation of meaningful options from which patients choose what is appropriate in consultation with nurses (Houston & Cowley 2002, Menon 2002).

# Partnership

As noted earlier in this chapter, there has been significant pressure to increase consumer participation in health care. Indeed, such participation has been endorsed and promoted by Australian health policy makers (Wellard et al 2003), and is enshrined in many policy documents. An increasing interest in partnership in patient–professional relationships is associated with this rise in consumerism, as well as legislation concerned with patients' rights, the women's movement and unexplained variations in doctors' practices (Charles et al 1999). The term 'partnership' has been defined as a relationship between individuals or groups that is characterised by mutual cooperation and responsibility for the achievement of a specified goal (Oxford Dictionary 2003).

In Chapter 2, Health, Wellness, Illness, Healing and Holism and Nursing, there is recognition of the therapeutic value of the nurse–patient relationship in collaboration and partnership. Chapter 2 explains that the healing partnership is grounded in a relationship where the nature of being human connects a nurse and patient. The term 'partnership' can mean different things to different people, so it is important to consider the underlying characteristics of a health care user and provider partnership.

These characteristics include non-patronising empowerment, collaborative decisions, valuing diversity and individuality and mutual benefit. Each of these is discussed in the next section, along with threats to each.

## Case study . . . *continued*

Three months have gone by and unfortunately Jim's condition has deteriorated. After discussions with his nurse at the Community Mental Health Clinic, Jim makes the decision to go to hospital. Peter visits him there, and is concerned to find his father visibly distressed and quite agitated.

P:  How are you going Dad?

J:  Not so great. I don't like it here.

P:  Why is that?

> J: I'm just here so they can pump me full of drugs and so all I do is sleep. No-one's talking to me.
>
> P: Have you talked to the nurses about this?
>
> J: What's the point? They'll just think I'm a crazy old fellow who doesn't know anything.

## Non-patronising empowerment

In health matters, empowerment is where the health care provider works alongside the health care consumer with a shared goal of enhanced health and wellbeing for the person receiving health care. This close relationship hinges on a sense of trust, respect, flexibility and reciprocal understanding. Nurses are very powerful in determining whether or not a truly empowering relationship is developed (Nyatanga & Dann 2002), since usually they must take the lead in setting up the right conditions for the partnership to thrive.

Despite the ideal, there are significant threats to the existence of an empowering relationship. These arise from the traditional perspective of health care, where nurses continue to hold stereotypical views of patients as passive recipients, where nurses claim professional authority, or where nurses may subtly manipulate or control the choices of those they care for. Jim experienced this subtle control by being excluded from discussion about his treatment once he was hospitalised. This stood in stark contrast to the ways in which he and his community mental health nurse had worked together. Perhaps his nurses in the acute mental health unit wanted Jim to have a few days of rest, to recover from the sleep deprivation he had been experiencing prior to hospitalisation and to adjust to his new medication regime. However, none of this was explained to him and so he felt excluded and devalued, and, most likely, very frightened. In Chapter 11, Journeys Through Illness: Suffering and Resilience, it was identified that suffering may be related to experiences of the care provided. It is not difficult to see that Jim was experiencing this kind of suffering.

### Case study . . . *continued*

Peter went to speak with the nursing staff about his father's concerns. The registered nurse caring for Jim immediately came to speak with him. She sat down next to Jim and expressed her concern that he was feeling so distressed. She asked him whether he would like to talk about how he felt, and he agreed. She listened quietly while he spoke. He told her that he was finding it hard to think at the moment, and he just wanted to know what was happening so that he could relax a bit. Once she ascertained that at that point Jim wanted to know more about his treatment regime, she spent some time discussing this with him. She was careful to speak clearly and without too much detail because she could see that Jim was struggling to remain alert. She suggested that they talk more in a few days time, when Jim was feeling better. Jim agreed, saying that he was feeling calmer.

## Collaborative decisions

Nurses and other health professionals have high levels of specialised knowledge, clinical expertise and professional experience. This knowledge, expertise and experience are most useful when combined with the wisdom that people who are ill have about their illness experience. Empowering of patients does not imply that nurses and other health professionals need to give up their professional power, but it does suggest that they are prepared to share that power by working alongside those they care for.

Many people with an illness are knowledgeable about their health problems. They may be active in support groups, read consciousness-raising books about health, and search the Internet for information. All these activities are self-empowering and, as a logical consequence, may well lead to the expectation of active involvement in decisions related to their health and health care. Individuals with chronic illness can develop sophisticated awareness of their body's patterns and responses that bear little resemblance to the textbook picture, but professionals are sometimes reluctant to acknowledge this expertise as credible (Paterson 2001).

The disciplinary education and training for many nurses may, in their mind, justify their expertise in making unilateral decisions. Nurses might argue that they must adhere to evidence-based practice, which means choosing health care interventions which have been demonstrated via research to be effective. They may be tempted to think that these interventions can be used without engaging in a collaborative decision-making process with those in their care. This approach has been criticised (Rogers 2002, p 99):

> [T]here is a lack of recognition that the production of such evidence is a complex process involving methodologically imposed limitations and value-laden decisions . . . The people making these decisions are clinicians, researchers, biostatisticians and epidemiologists rather than patients, so that the results of systematic reviews may not necessarily reflect the outcomes of interest to patients.

Empowering partnerships do not take 'power' from one to give to another. Instead, they create a symbiosis that produces a greater and more helpful caring process than either the carer or the person in care can do individually (McKay et al 1990, p 86). The shared wisdom made possible through collaborative decision making is holistic in nature because, as suggested in Chapter 2, a holistic approach implies something more than the sum of its parts.

### Case study . . . *continued*

Peter regularly visited his father in hospital. After two weeks, Jim was feeling well enough to think about going home.

J: It's been quite a learning curve, this whole hospital business.

P: I'll bet.

J:   I was happy to do what I was told early on, once they explained what they were doing. But now I'm feeling better, and I want to make my own decisions. Sure they're kind, and they know a lot, but it's me that's got to deal with this thing. They can't really feel what I feel, even though I've tried to tell them. First thing I want to do when I get home is to get on the Internet. Apparently there are some real good discussion groups for people with depression. I reckon that could really help. I'm going back to that nurse at the clinic. He's good. Still he can't do it for me. I've got to look after myself.

## Valuing diversity and individuality

Valuing the diversity and individuality of each health care user requires a recognition of the uniqueness of that person, as well as an appreciation that that person is the expert with regard to his/her life situation. There is a potential pitfall, however, in assuming that all patients want a collaborative partnership. Some have argued that patients must be active and equal participants in their own empowerment (Kuokkanen & Leino-Kilpi 2000) but this sounds very much like an imposed value.

Some people will want to be in full control of their health care and make all decisions, whilst others may want to be given information and directive advice about the best options. Jim was decisive in that he wanted to be included in discussion about his health care needs and treatment but this is not always the case. Others will prefer that control remains with their health care providers, whom they see as the experts best able to make the right decisions. However the latter does not give nurses an inherent right to be in control of all decisions without regard to the person's situation.

This does not mean that if a health care user's choice might be detrimental to their health that the nurse stands back and does nothing. Nurses have a duty of care to counsel those they care for about the choices they are making. The collectiveness of a partnership is about coming together, valuing the expertise of each other and gaining more by working collaboratively and in partnership than if acting alone. So, in the cases where the choice made will adversely affect the health care user, it is advised that the nurse discuss the issues with the aim of assisting the health care user to make a choice based on a shared perspective. This approach by the health carer best fulfils the moral sense of benevolent concern (Woodward 1998).

Unrealistic workload and the deeply embedded tradition of routine and task orientation of nurses present a threat to facilitating choice and individualised care. The demands on nurses' time and resources might make them susceptible to deciding what is best for the health care users, which then might lead to the imposition of their own values, thereby establishing a paternalistic approach, rather than a partnership. Other threats to valuing diversity and individuality may be exposed if nurses are unable to take into account the characteristics of each person, such as gender, age, ethnicity, and regional location, as discussed in previous chapters.

> ## Case study . . . *continued*
>
> Peter caught up with the registered nurse (RN) who talked with his father. She was pleased to have done that.
>
> RN: I am really grateful that we became aware of your father's concerns. We get so used to our own routine that we can easily forget that our patients don't know what's going on.
>
> P: Yes I know. I fall into that trap myself. We're always so busy; and sometimes it just feels that you've got to get on with the work and I guess the 'niceties' get lost.
>
> RN: Yes, but you know what? Jim was so much easier to care for once he felt like we were working with him. Once I'd explained everything, and given him some options, his agitation settled and he helped us out, rather than fighting against us. We saved more time in the long run!

# Mutual benefit

A partnership relationship between health care users and providers is mutually beneficial as the shared experience enriches the lives of both learners and teachers to each other. This benefit is exponentially increased because the providers' enriched expertise and experience serve them well in their next partnerships. For the health care users, an empowering partnership provides a sense of being able to influence their own state of health, a sense of self-efficacy in effecting their own accomplishments and an appreciation for their abilities (Pretty 1998).

For nurses there is a strong connection, identification and a sense of being a part of the journey with that health care user, where presence is more than a physical attendance. A real sense of satisfaction can derive from that experience (Parker 2001, p 90):

> We become autonomous through engagement with others, through being taught and through learning, through being offered choice and through offering them to others.

Yet, health care professionals still experience difficulty in relinquishing control (Waterworth & Lucker 1990, Jewell 1996). Some reasons offered as explanation for this are:

- the hierarchy and predominantly authoritarian interactional style, in professions such as nursing (Nyatanga & Dann 2002);
- reluctance of professionals to acknowledge the expertise of health care consumers (Paterson 2001);
- communication styles (Keating et al 2002);
- professional style (Wellard et al 2003); and
- environmental constraints (Wellard et al 2003).

Perhaps a positive way to frame a move to supportive, empowering partnerships between nurses and users is to first acknowledge the differing expertise that both can bring to the partnership itself.

## Conclusion

The existence of a relationship between a health care user and nurse does not automatically equate to a partnership. As discussed in this chapter, a partnership is both a structure and process, where two or more people share power and negotiate ways in which to obtain the mutually agreed goals. The health care user has individualised and unique knowledge and experience of their situation, including managing symptoms and daily adapting or accommodating their illness, whilst the nurse has knowledge of the disease, illness and management as it relates to the general population. Thus 'the collective strengths of the partners can enrich the definition of respective roles and responsibilities as well as outcomes of the partnership' (Gallant et al 2002, p 153).

This book has focused on the different aspects of the experience of illness and challenges nurses to move beyond a single, biomedical orientation to the delivery of nursing care. People accessing health care have a wide, diverse and rich range of experiences and expertise that, when brought into a collaborative and supportive partnership with their nurses, provides an environment that truly offers and supports a holistic approach in the provision of nursing care.

## Tutorial questions

1. Our personal beliefs about the relationship between those we care for and ourselves as their nurses will influence our nursing practice. What are your beliefs abut nurse–client relationships? To what extent do your beliefs fit within an empowering partnership model?
2. What are the characteristics or vulnerabilities of each of the following groups which may prevent them from being active participants in empowering partnerships with the nurses who care for them:
    a) immigrants;
    b) the elderly;
    c) those experiencing pain; and
    d) those from rural or remote areas.
3. What are the key aspects of an empowering relationship? What strategies will you use to develop empowering relationships with those you care for?

## References

Charles C, Whelan T, Gafni A 1999 What do we mean by partnership in making decisions about treatment? *British Medical Journal* 319:780–782

Gallant MH, Beaulieu MC, Carnevale FA 2002 Partnership: an analysis of the concept within the nurse-client relationship. *Journal of Advanced Nursing* 402:149–157

Germov J 1999 Challenges to medical dominance. In: Germov J (ed), *Second Opinion: An Introduction to Health Sociology* (revised edn). Oxford University Press, Melbourne, pp 230–248

Houston AM, Cowley S 2002 An empowerment approach to needs assessment in health visiting practice. *Journal of Clinical Nursing* 11:640–650

Jewell SE 1996 Elderly patients' participation in discharge decision making. *British Journal of Nursing* 5:914–932

Keating D, Bellchambers H, Bujack E, Cholowski K, Conway J, Neal P 2002 Communication: principal barrier to nurse-consumer partnerships. *International Journal of Nursing Practice* 8:16–22

Kuokkanen L, Leino-Kilpi H 2000 Power and empowerment in nursing: three theoretical approaches. *Journal of Advanced Nursing* 31(1):235–241

McKay B, Forbes JA, Bourner K 1990 Empowerment in general practice: the trilogies of caring. *Australian Family Physician* 19:513–520

McQueen A 2000 Nurse–patient relationships and partnership in hospital care. *Journal of Clinical Nursing* 9:723–731

Menon ST 2002 Toward a model of psychological health empowerment: implications for health care in multicultural communities. *Nurse Education Today* 22:28–39

Nyatanga L, Dann KL 2002 Empowerment in nursing: the role of philosophical and psychological factors. *Nursing Philosophy* 3:234–239

Oxford Dictionary 2003, Oxford University Press, Oxford

Parker M 2001 The ethics of evidence-based patient choice. *Health Expectations* 4:87–91

Parsons T 1950 The Social System. Free Press, New York

Paterson B 2001 Myth of empowerment in chronic illness. *Journal of Advanced Nursing* 34(5):574–581

Pretty G 1998 Woman Caring for Herself. In: Rogers-Clark C, Smith A (eds) *Women's Health: A Primary Health Care Approach*. MacLennan and Petty, Sydney, pp 19–33

Rogers WA 2002 Evidence-based medicine in practice: Limiting or facilitating patient choice? *Health Expectations* 5:95–103

Ryles SM 1999 A concept analysis of empowerment: its relationship to mental health nursing. *Journal of Advanced Nursing* 29(3):600–607

Tanner D 1998 Empowerment and care management: swimming against the tide. *Health and Social Care in the Community* 6(6) 447–457

Waterworth S, Lucker KA 1990 Reluctant collaborators: do patients want to be involved in decisions concerning care? *Journal of Advanced Nursing* 15:971–976

Watt S 2000 Clinical decision-making in the context of chronic illness. *Health Expectations* 3:6–16

Wellard S, Lillibridge J, Beanland C, Lewis M 2003 Consumer participation in acute care settings: an Australian experience. *International Journal of Nursing Practice* 9:255–260

Woodward VM 1998 Caring, patient autonomy and the stigma of paternalism. *Journal of Advanced Nursing* 28(5)1046–1052

# Index